Suck It Breast Cancer Coloring Book

Color Test Page

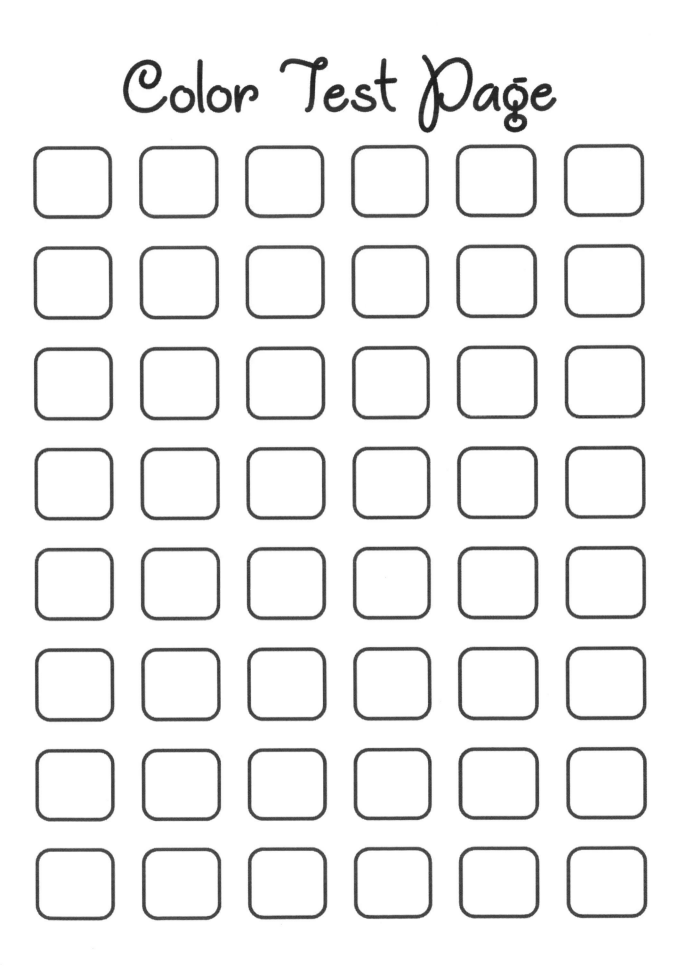

Color Test Page

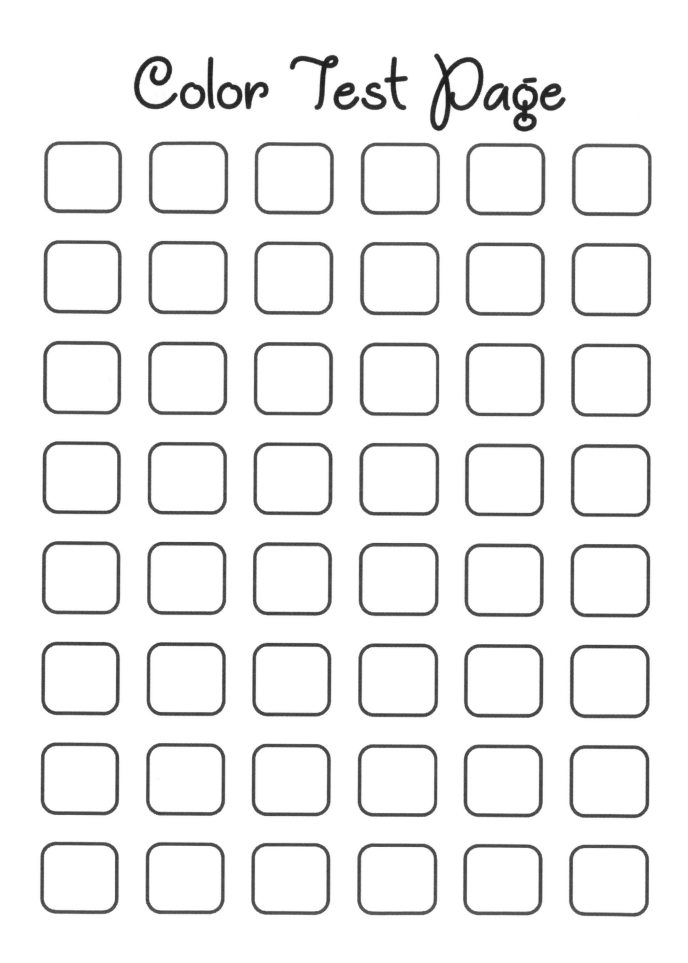

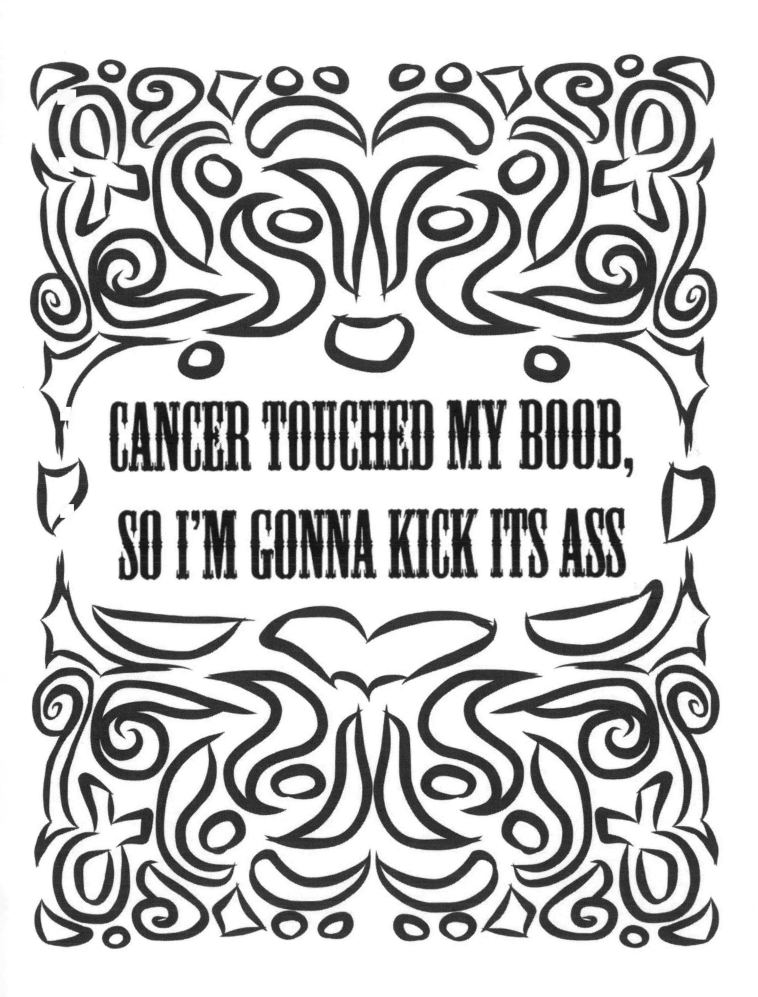

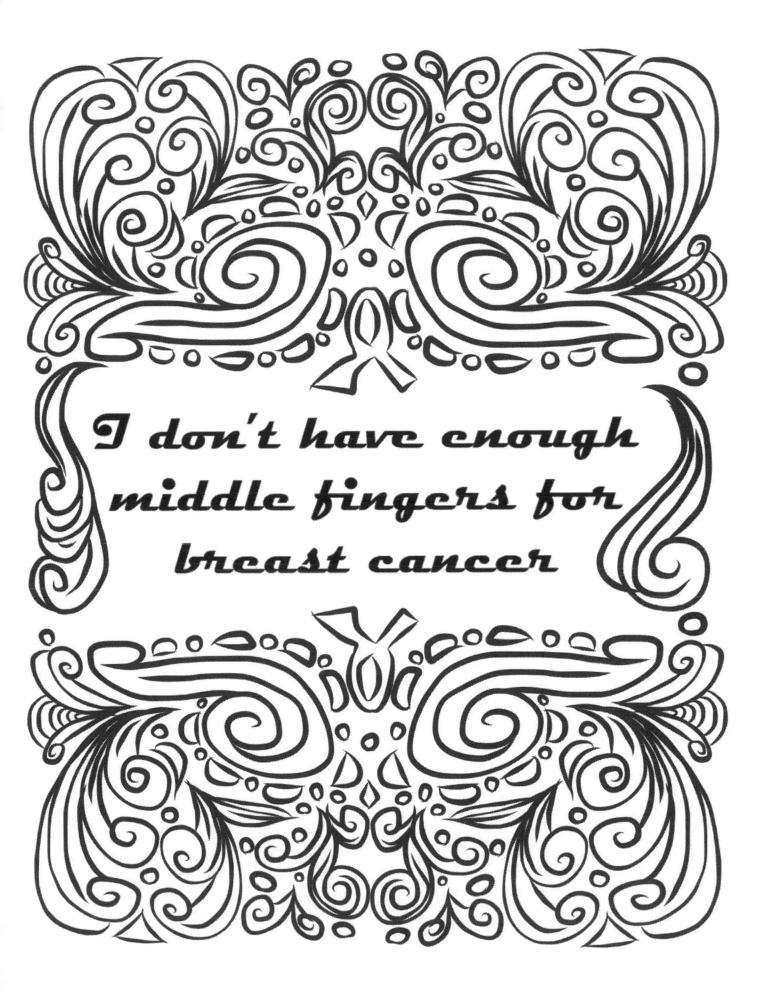

I don't have enough middle fingers for breast cancer

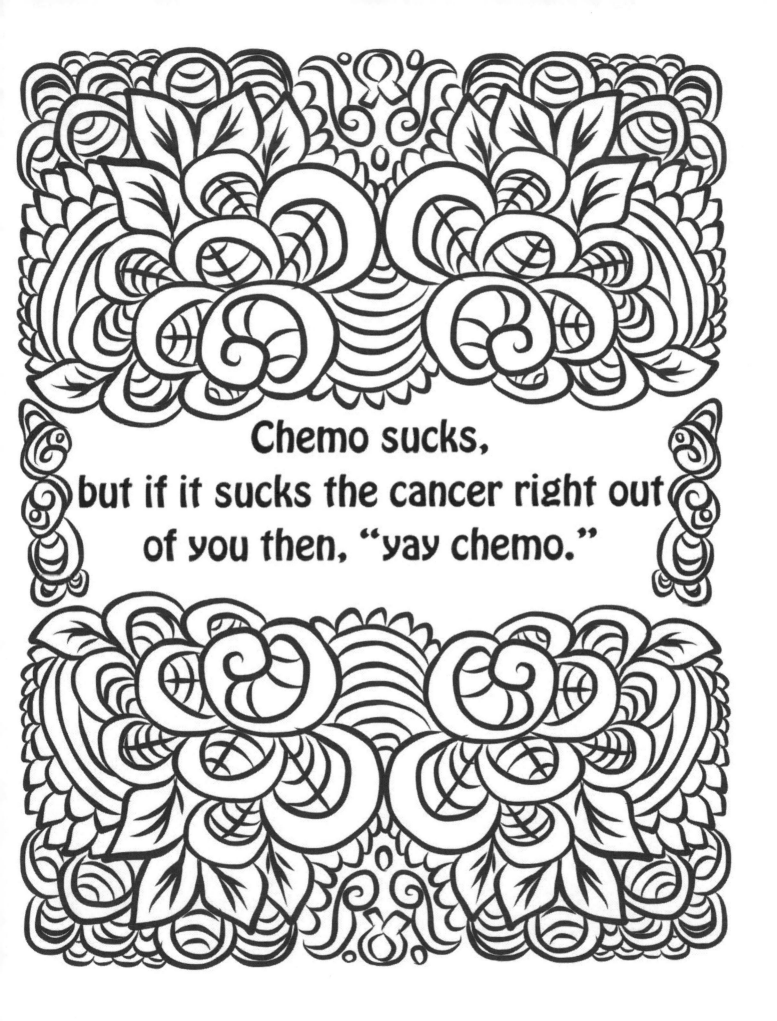

Chemo sucks,
but if it sucks the cancer right out
of you then, "yay chemo."

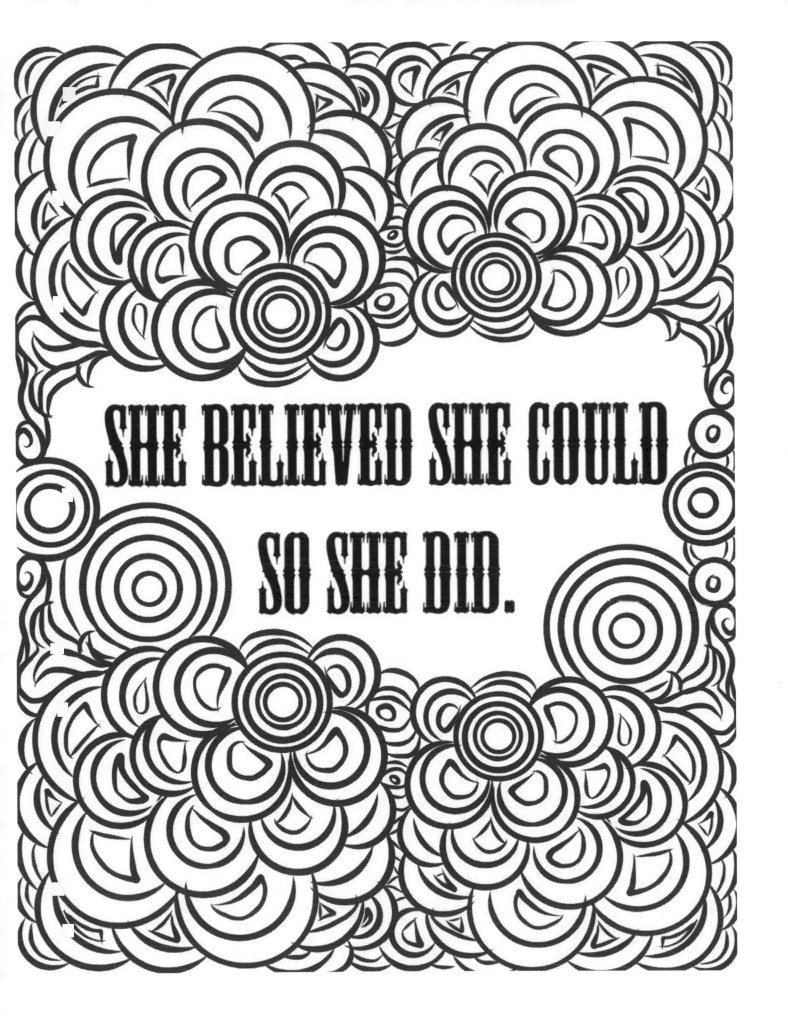

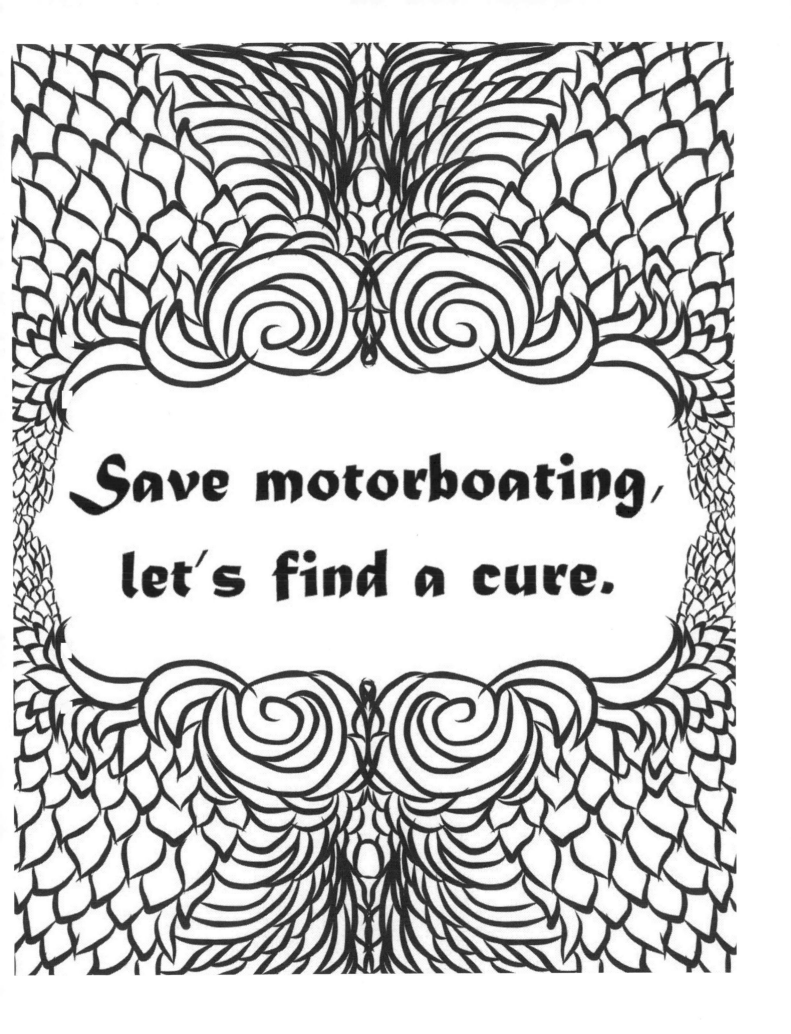

Save motorboating, let's find a cure.

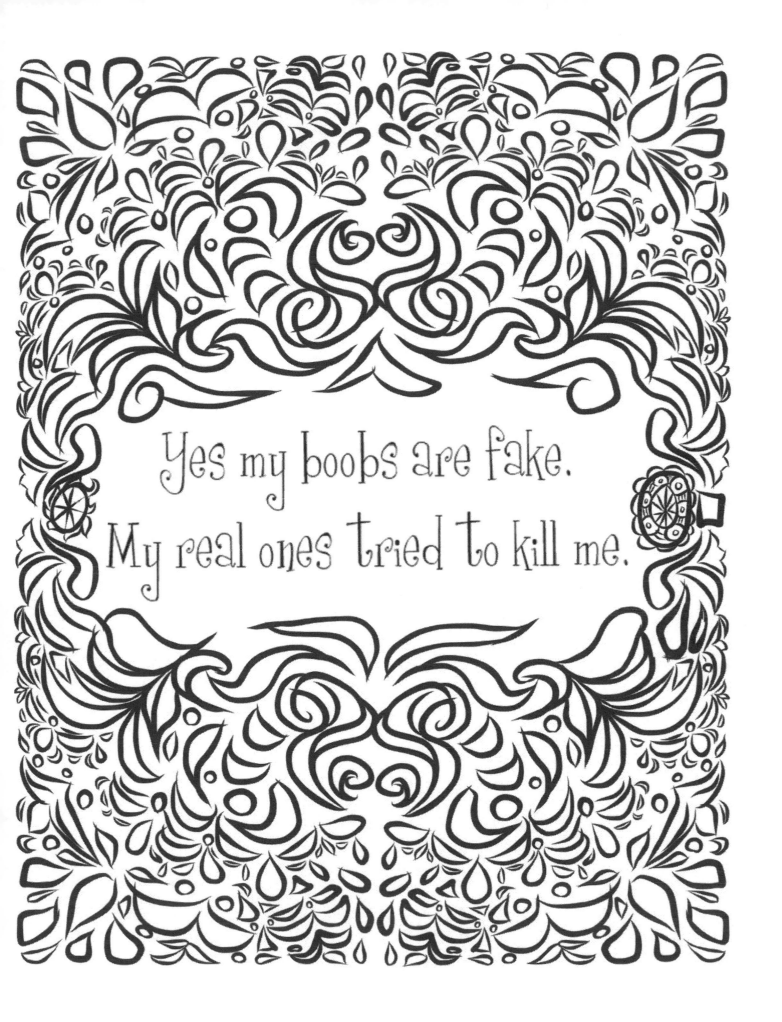

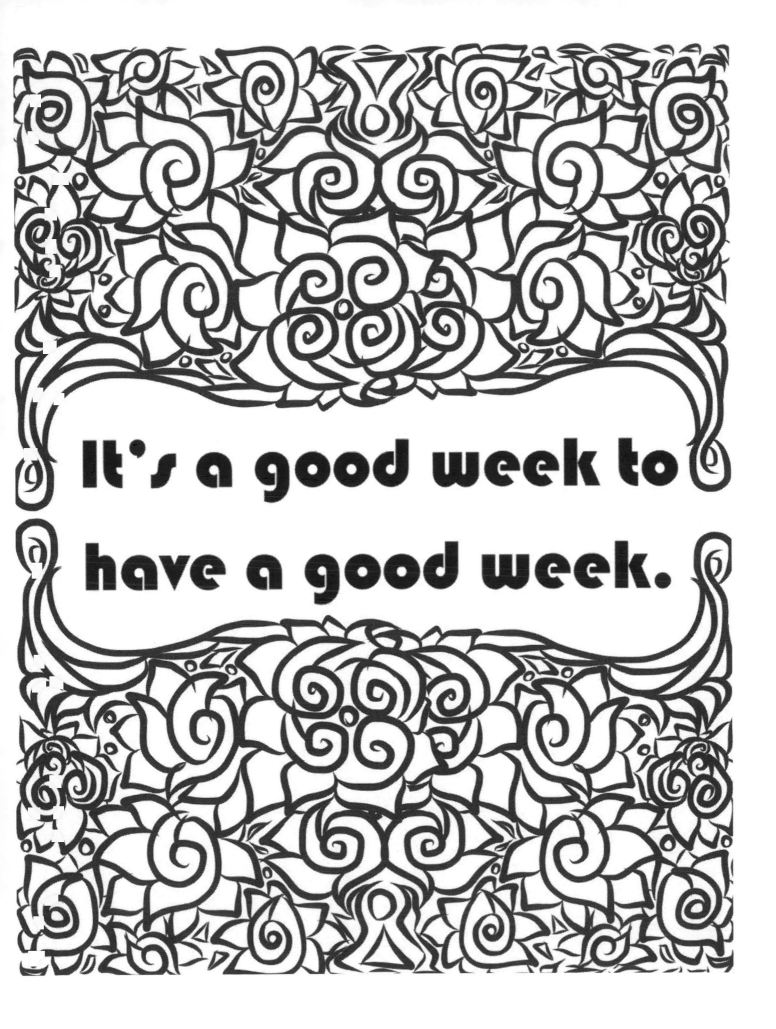

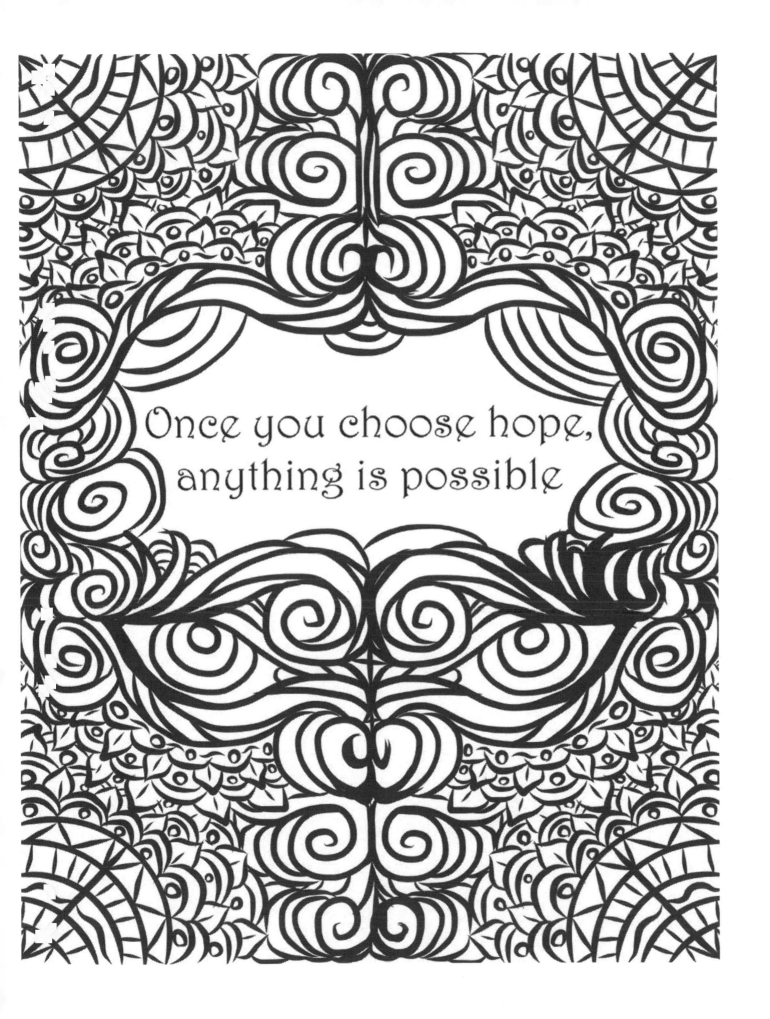

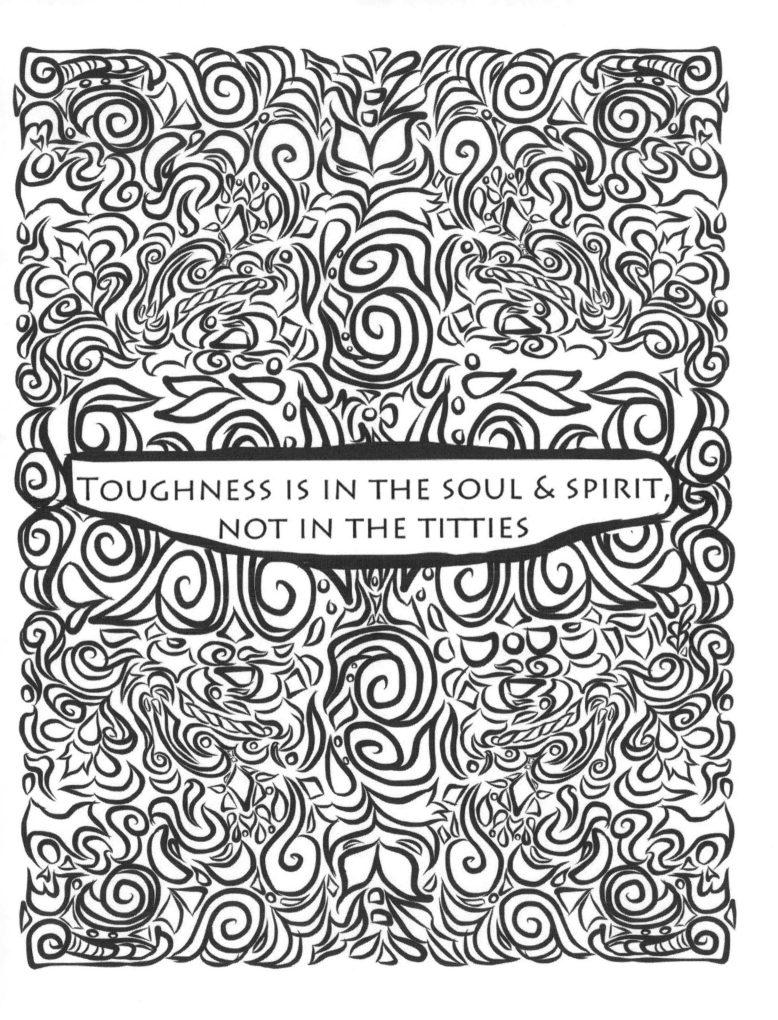

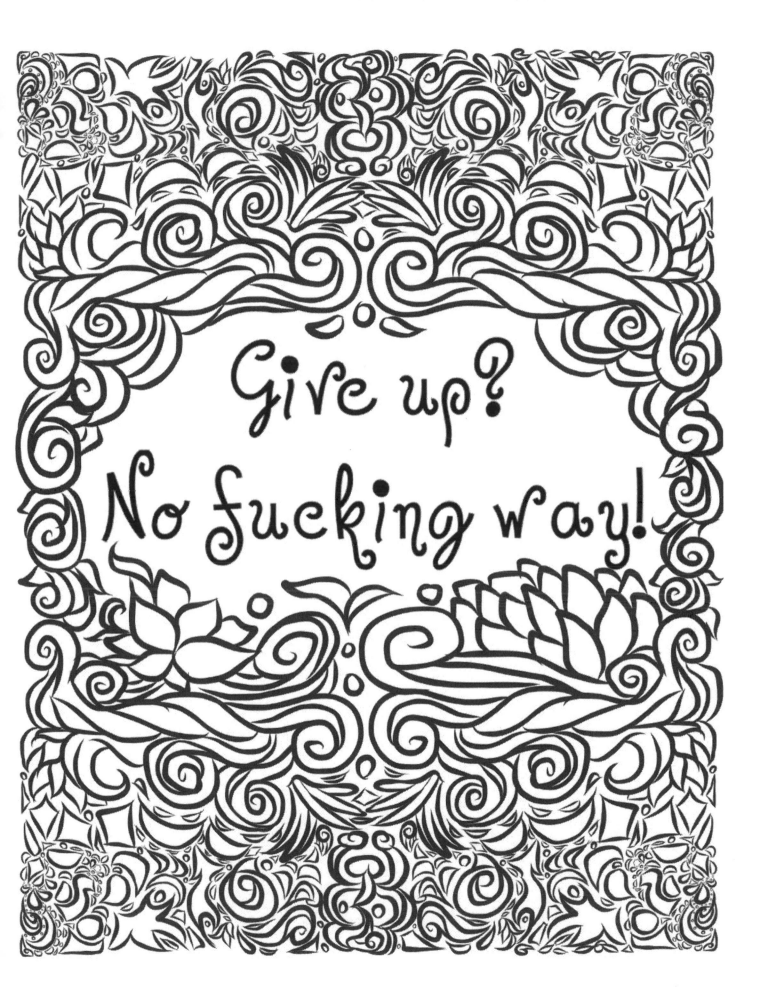

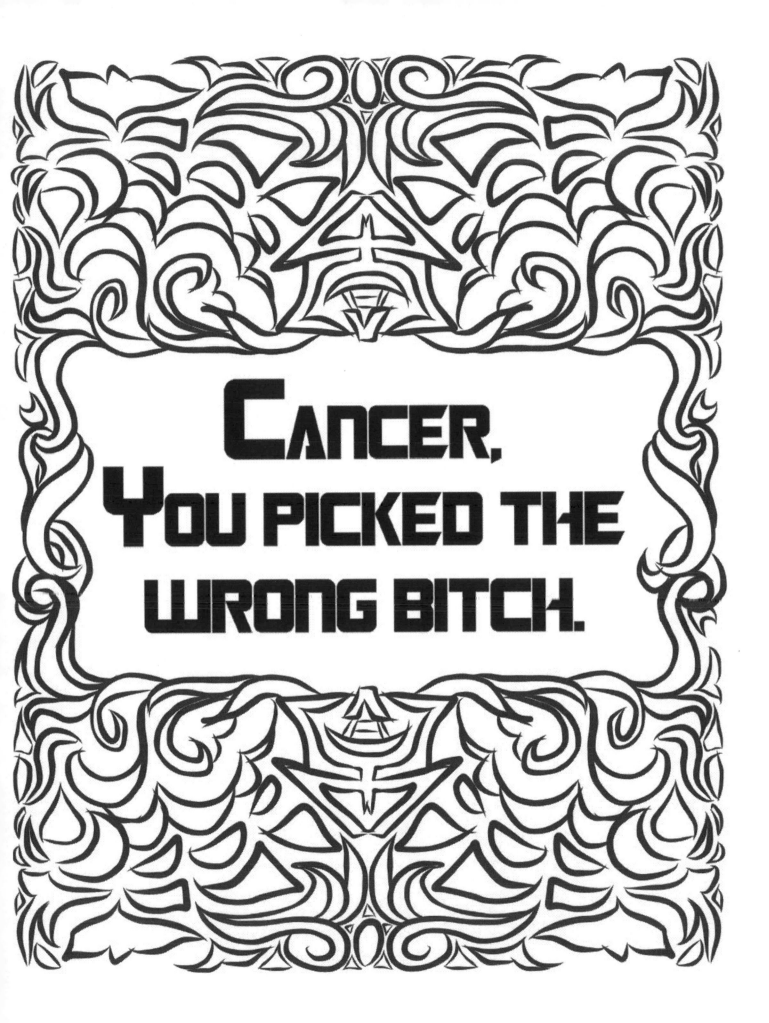

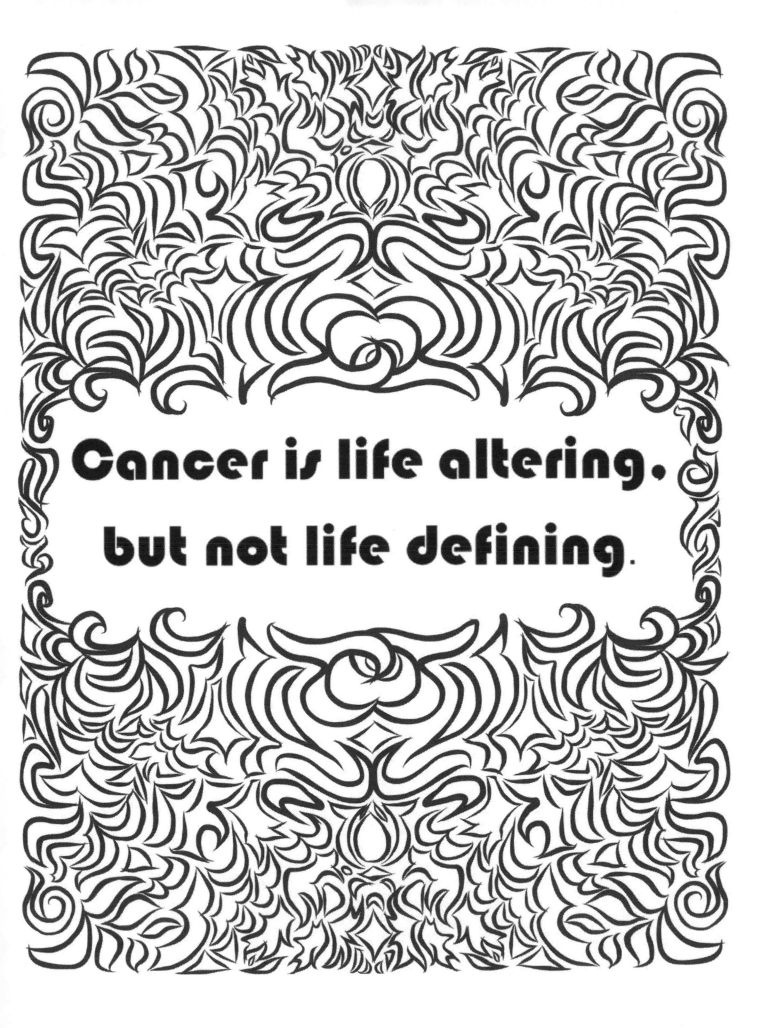

Cancer is life altering, but not life defining.

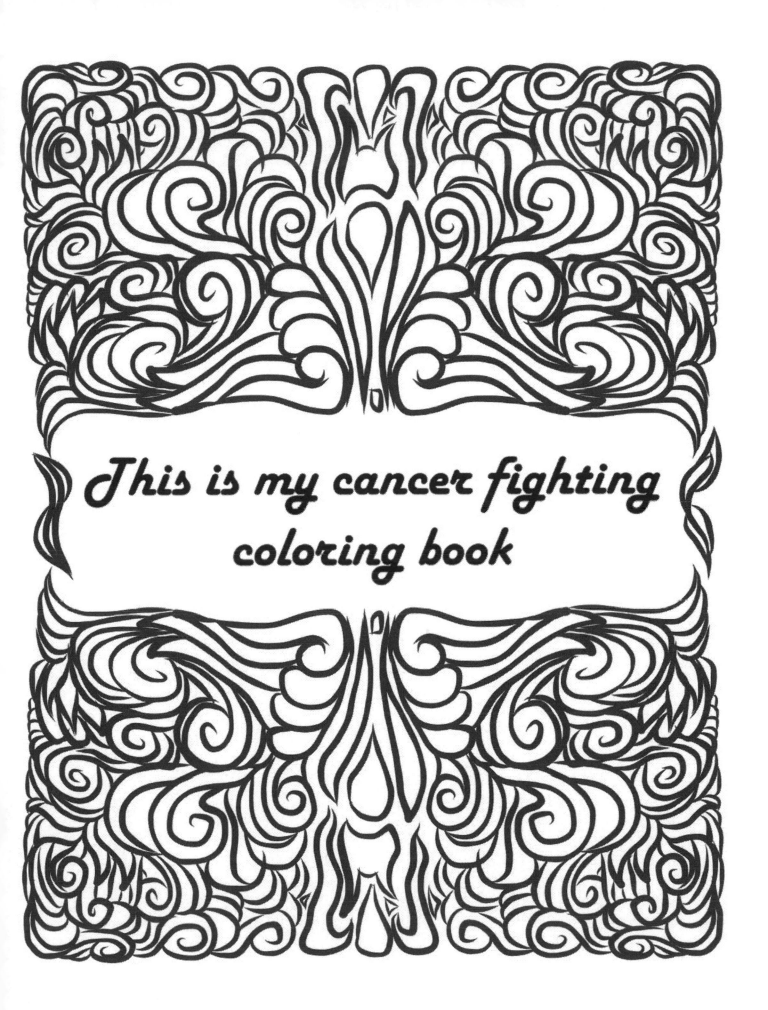

This is my cancer fighting coloring book

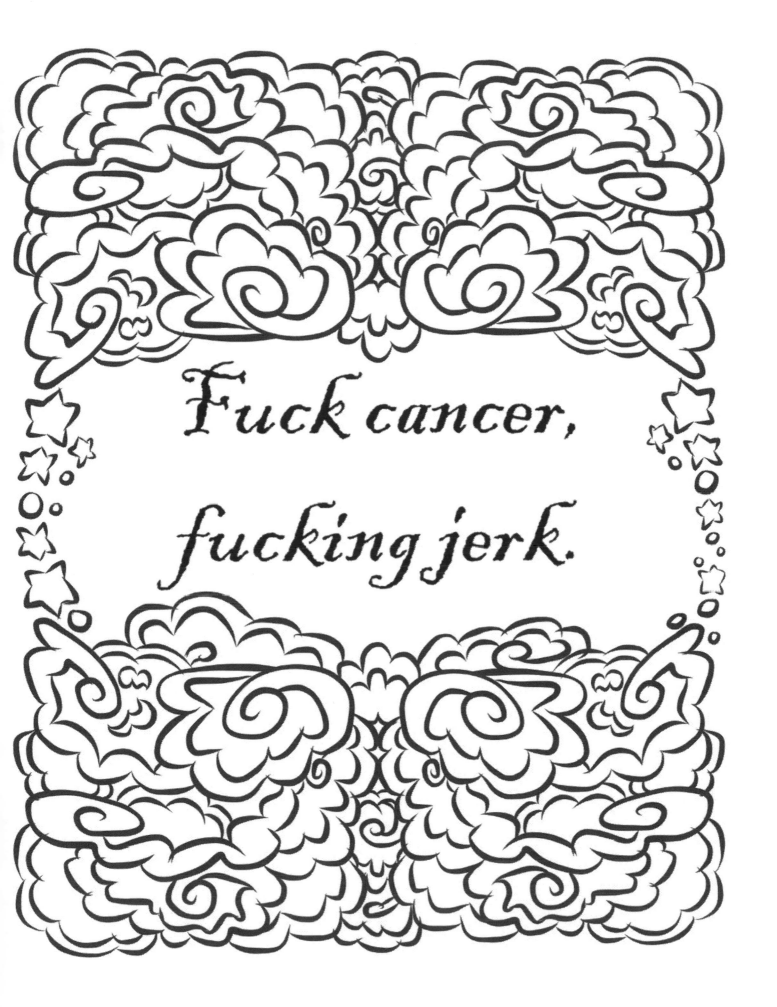

Fuck cancer,

fucking jerk.

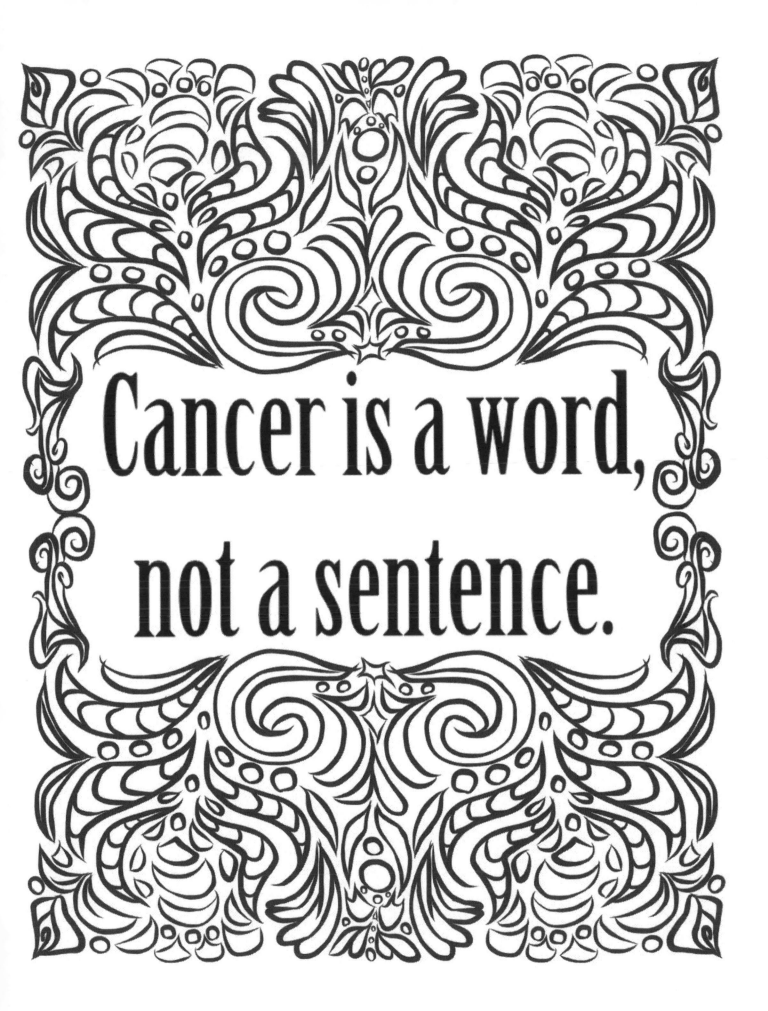

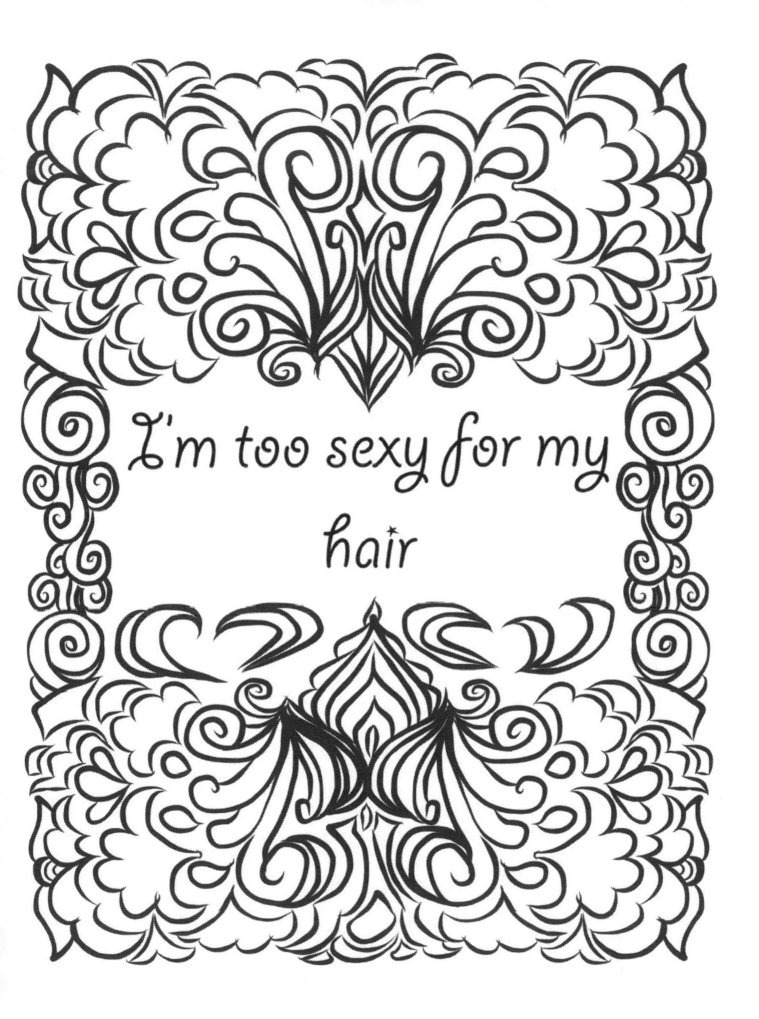

I'm too sexy for my hair

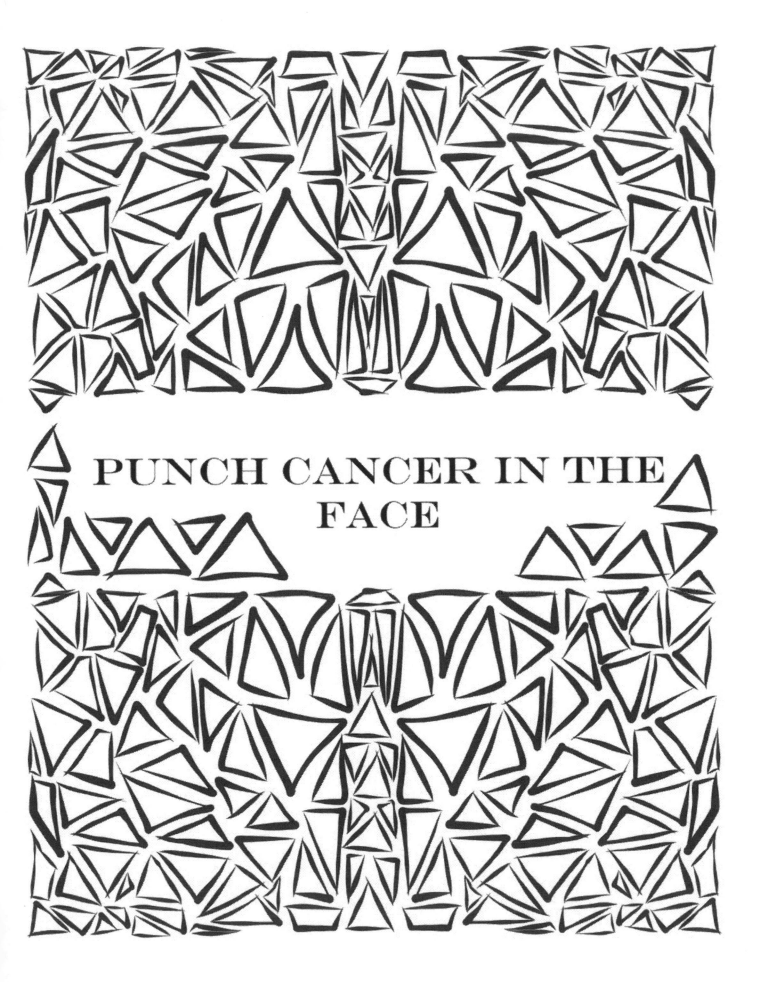

PUNCH CANCER IN THE
FACE

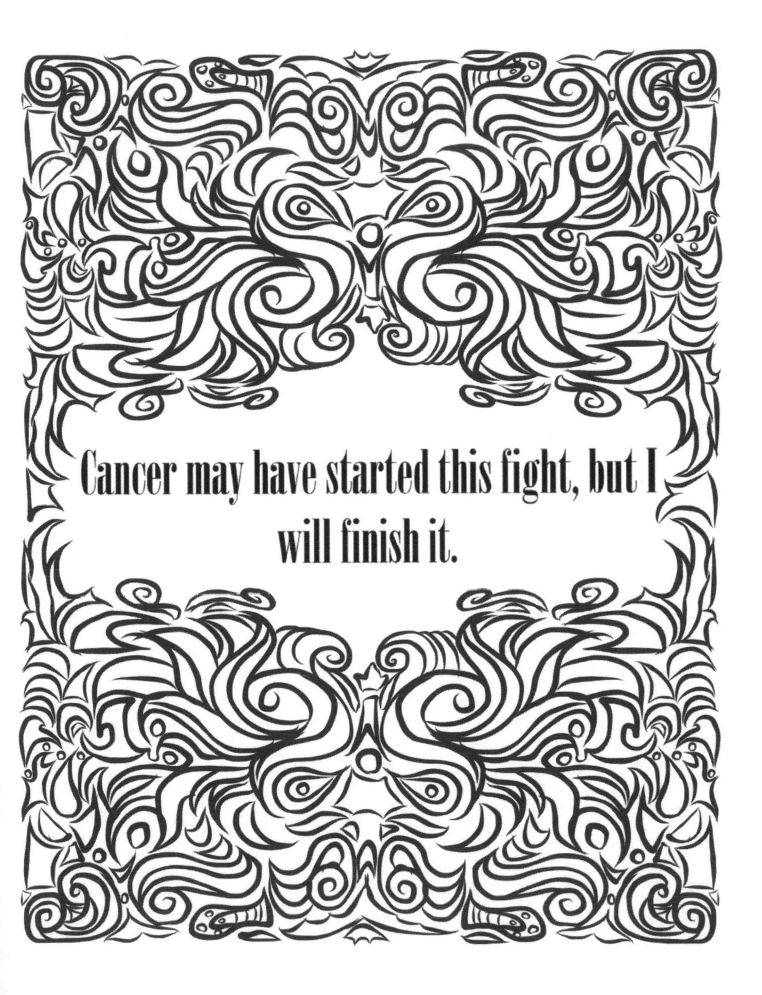

Cancer may have started this fight, but I will finish it.

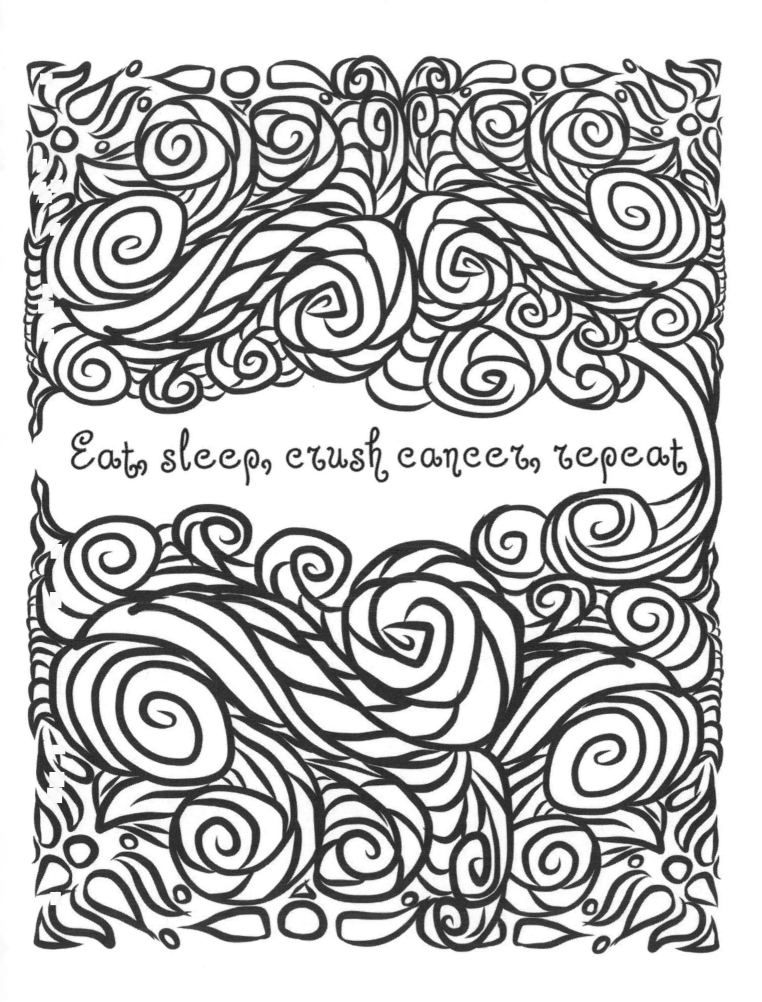

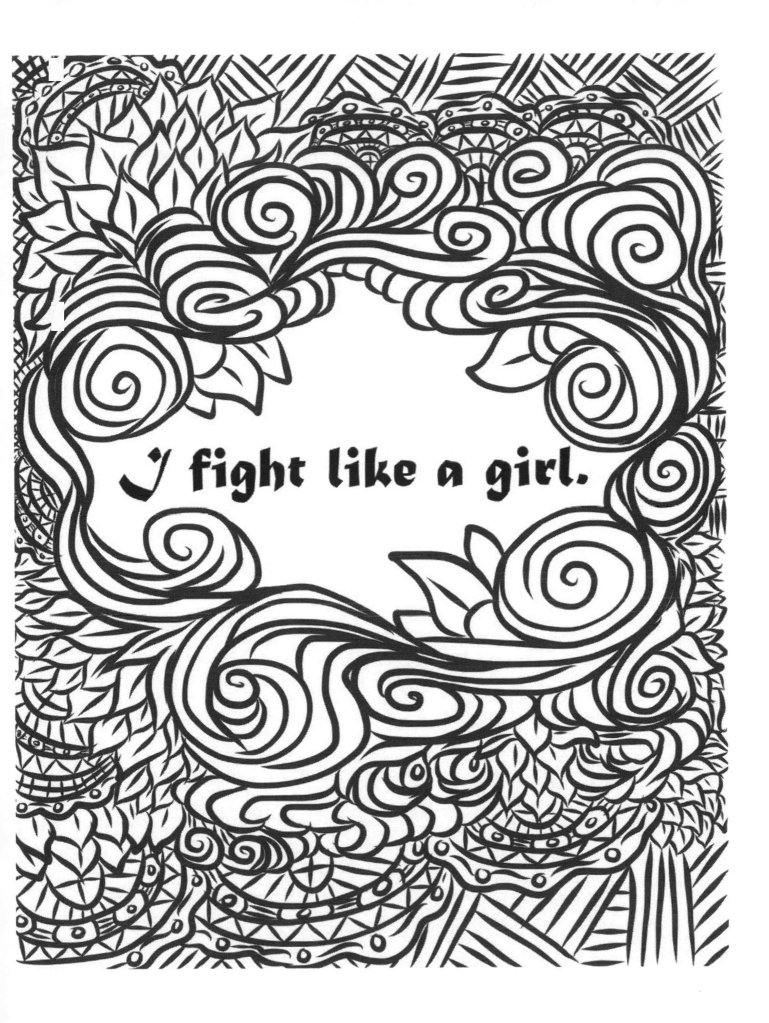

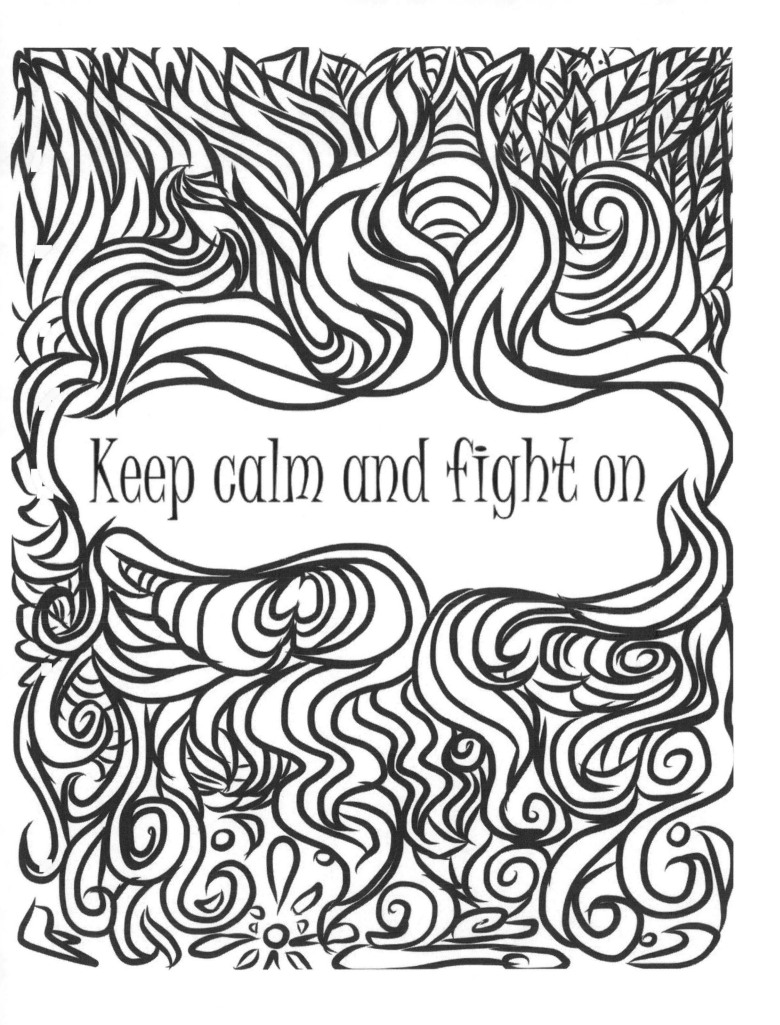

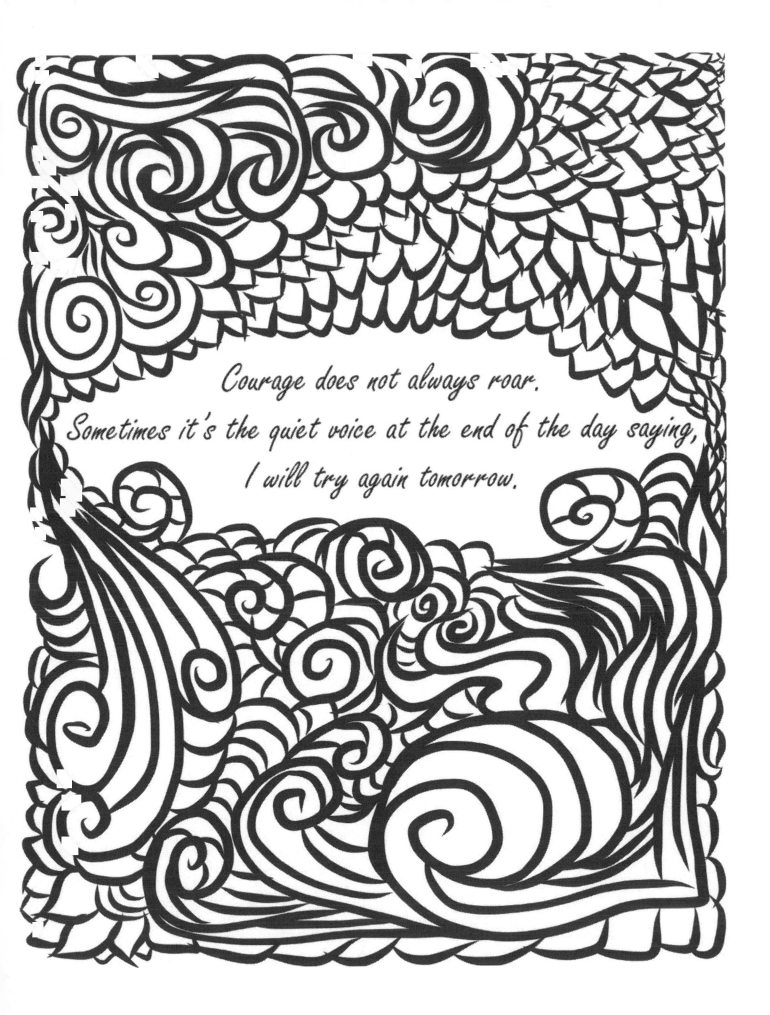

Courage does not always roar.

Sometimes it's the quiet voice at the end of the day saying,

I will try again tomorrow.

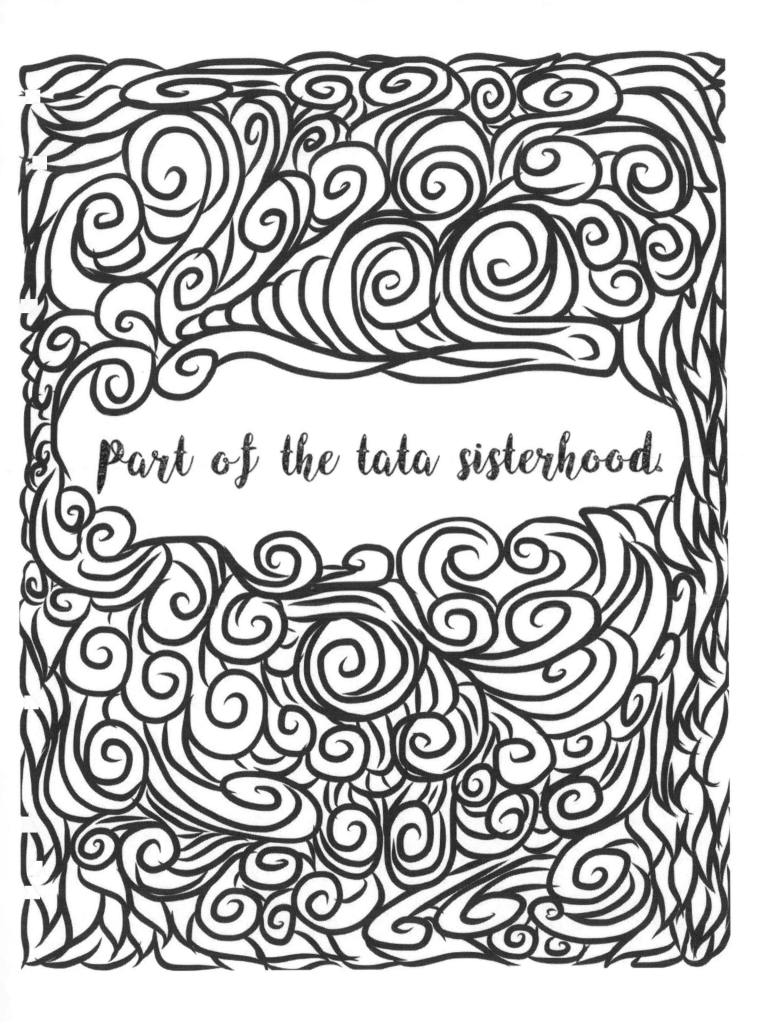

part of the tata sisterhood

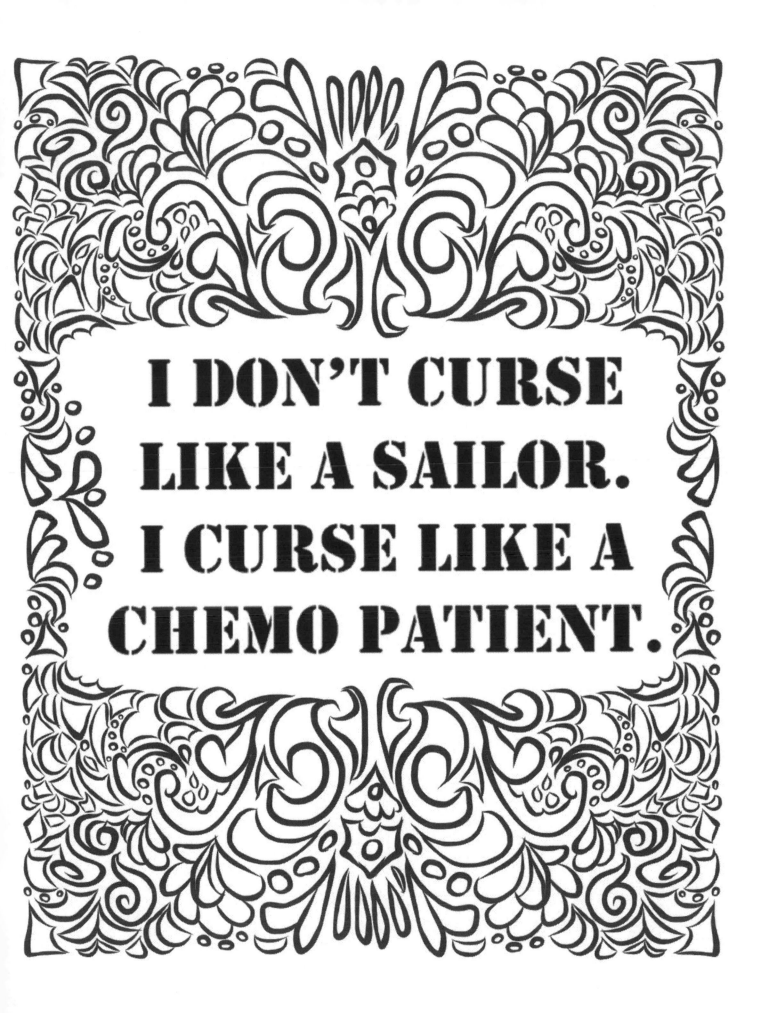

I AM NOT WHAT HAPPENED TO ME.
I AM WHAT I CHOOSE TO BECOME.

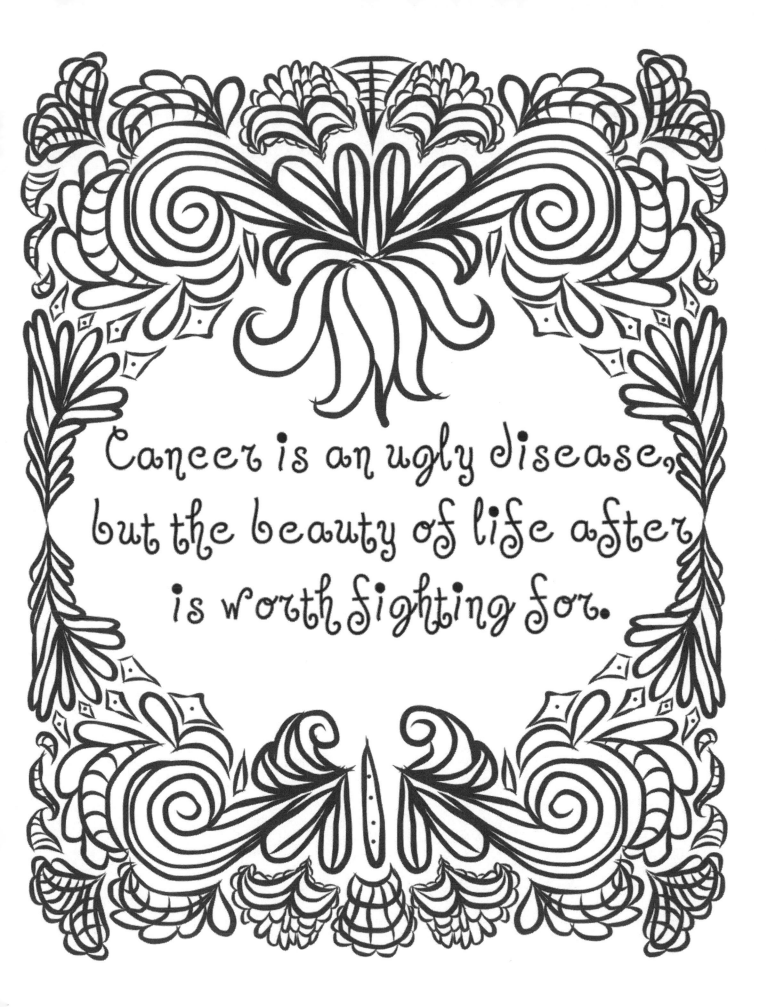

Cancer is an ugly disease, but the beauty of life after is worth fighting for.

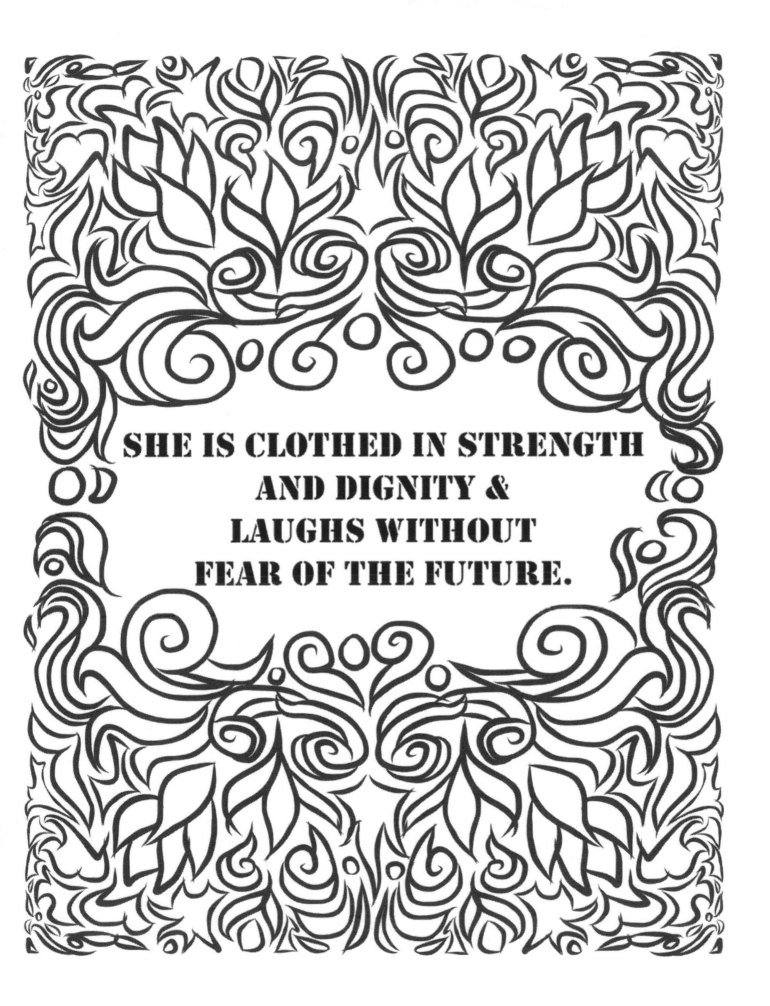

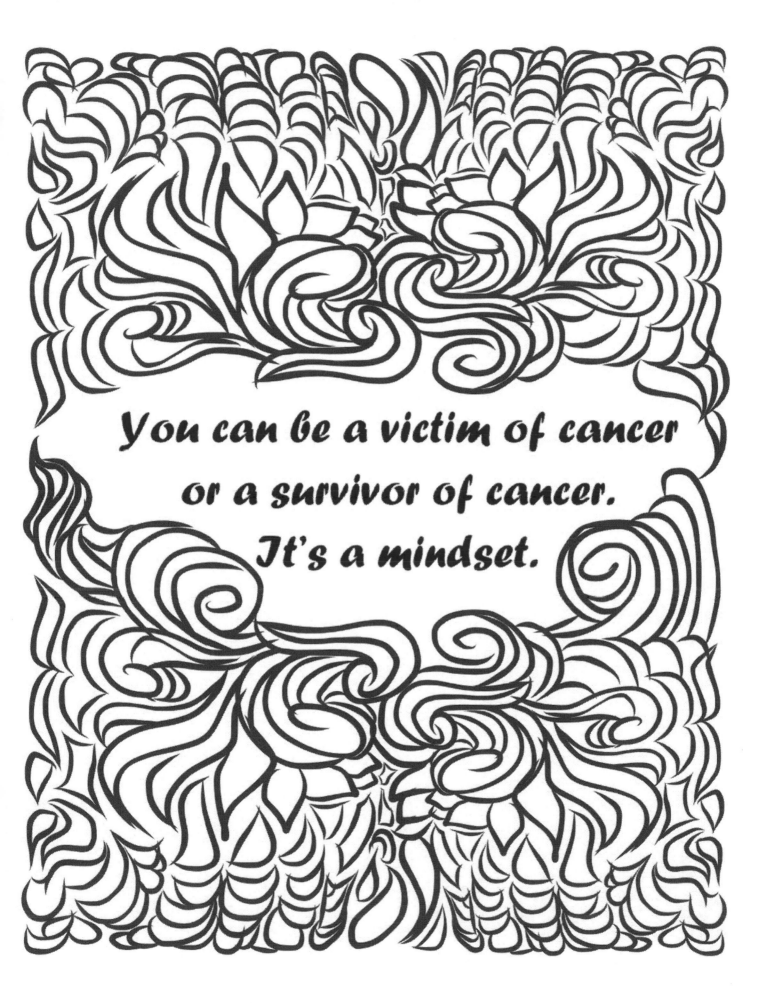

You can be a victim of cancer or a survivor of cancer. It's a mindset.

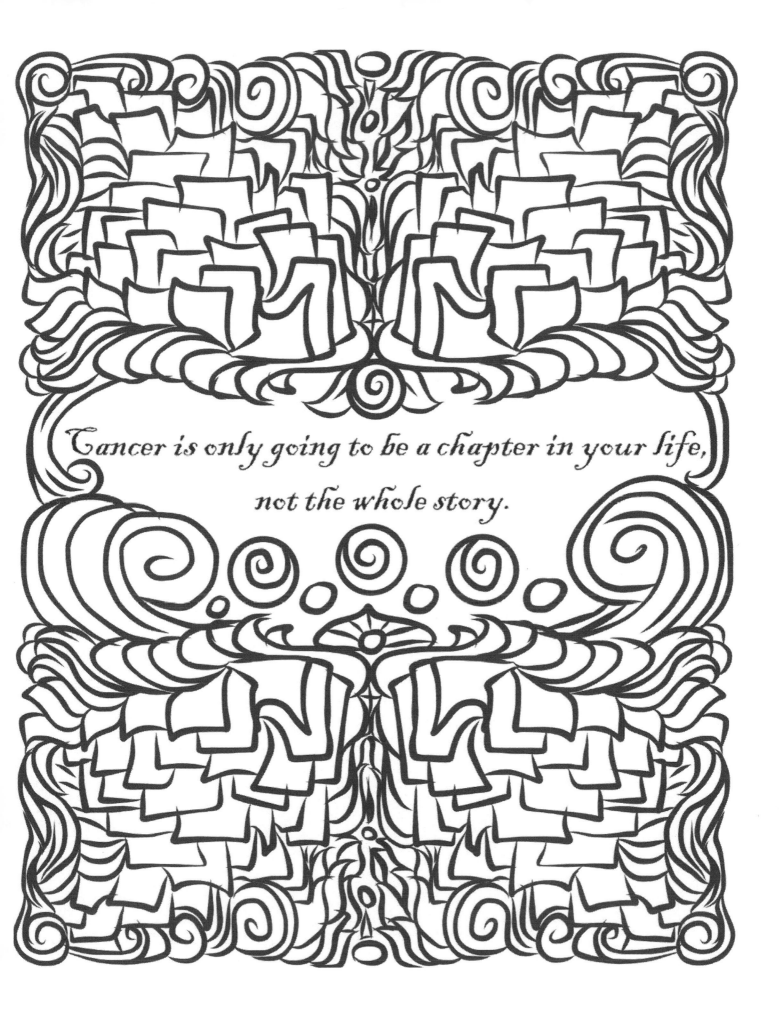

Cancer is only going to be a chapter in your life,

not the whole story.

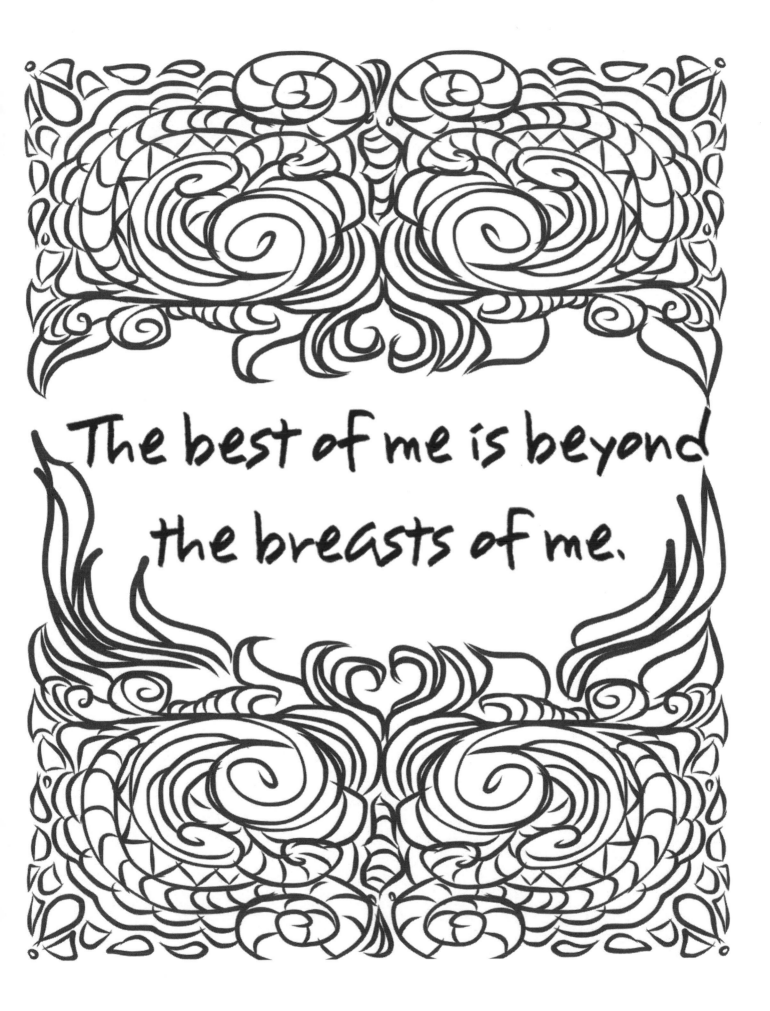

The best of me is beyond
the breasts of me.

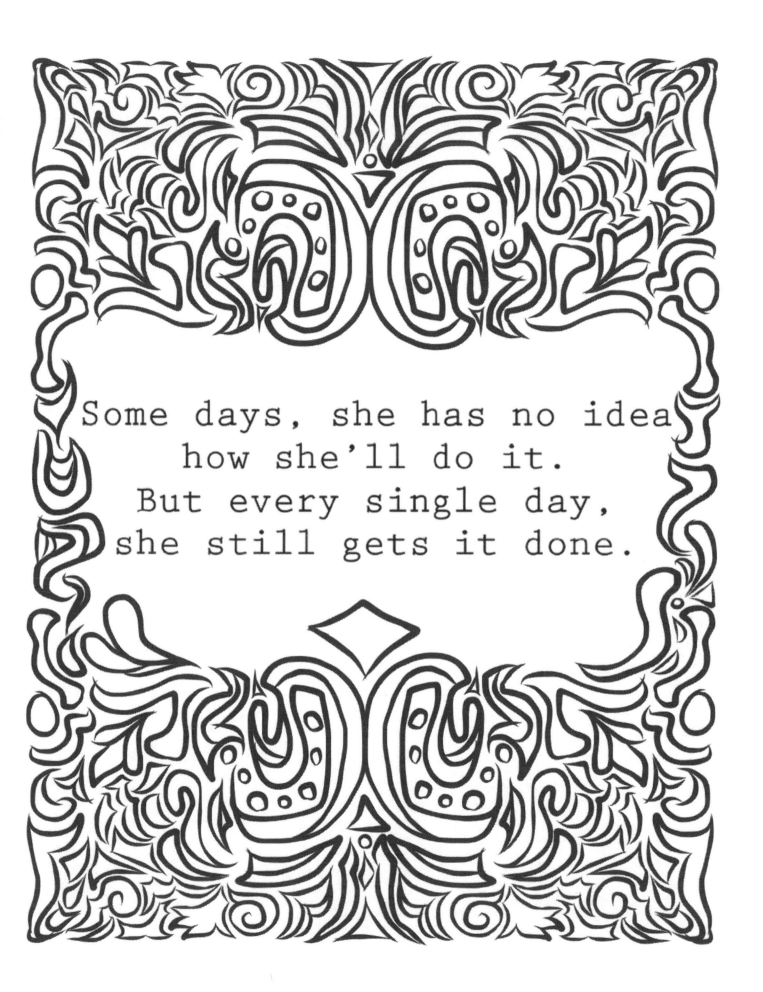

Some days, she has no idea
how she'll do it.
But every single day,
she still gets it done.

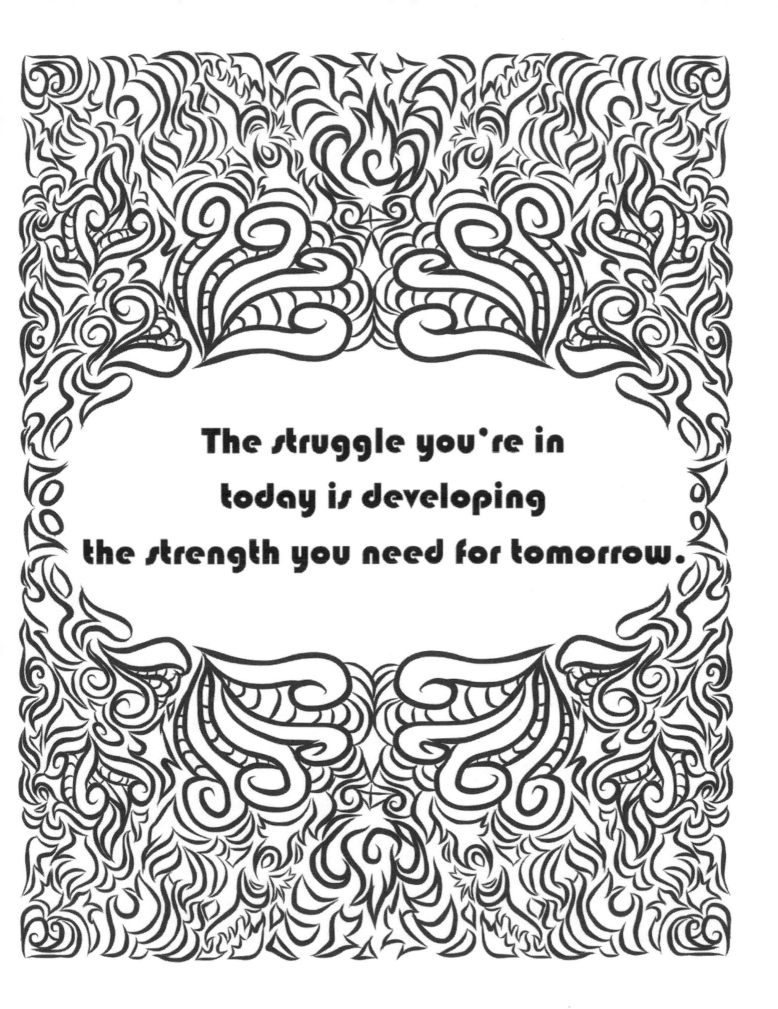

The struggle you're in today is developing the strength you need for tomorrow.

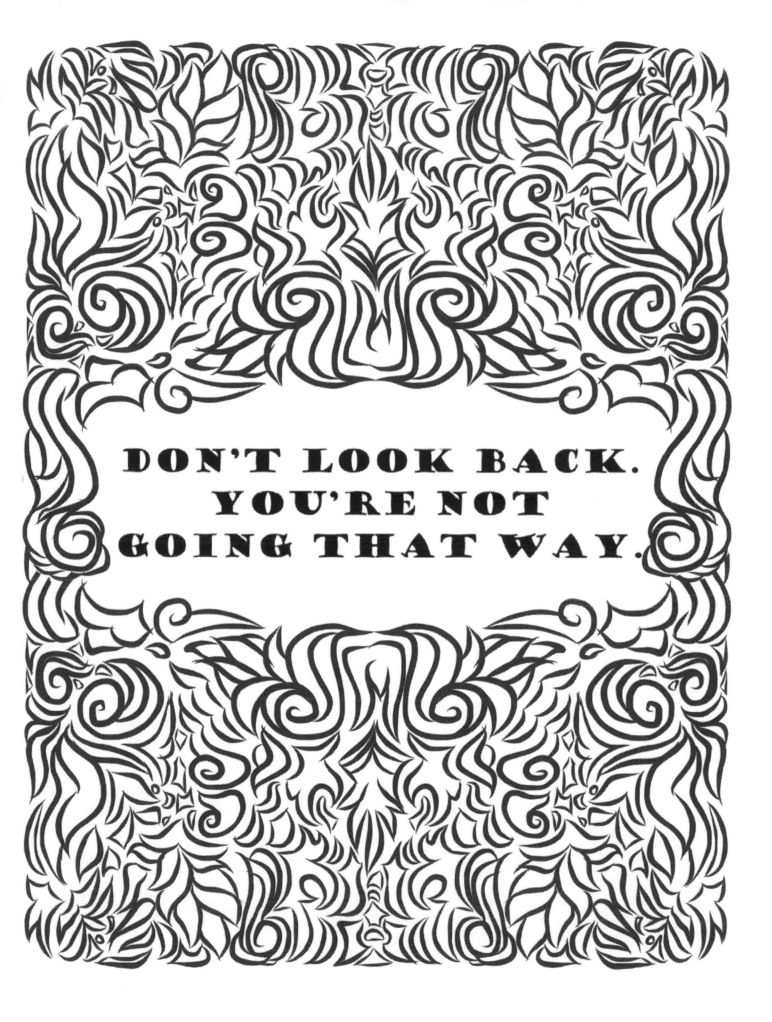

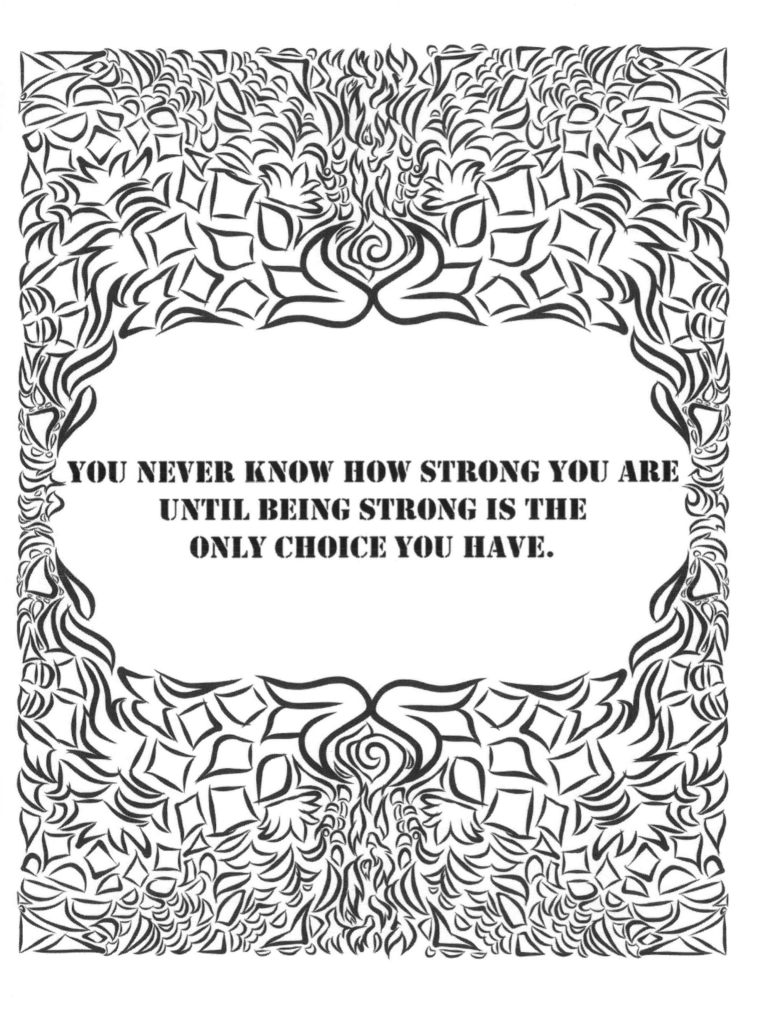

YOU NEVER KNOW HOW STRONG YOU ARE
UNTIL BEING STRONG IS THE
ONLY CHOICE YOU HAVE.

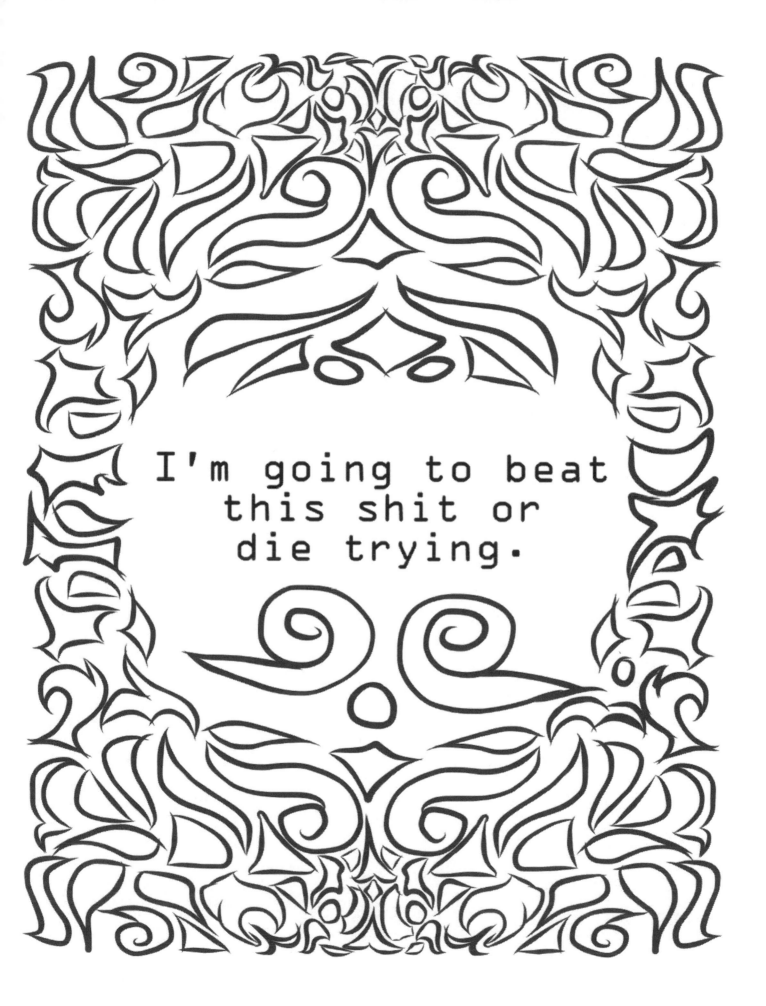

I'm going to beat
this shit or
die trying.

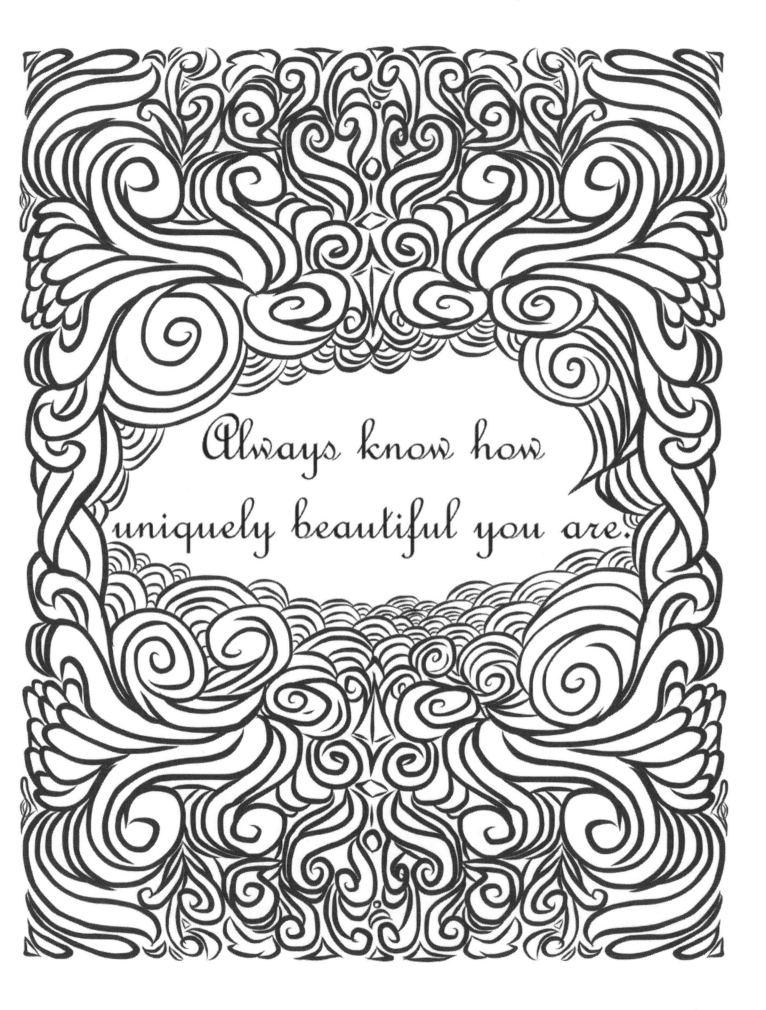

Always know how uniquely beautiful you are.

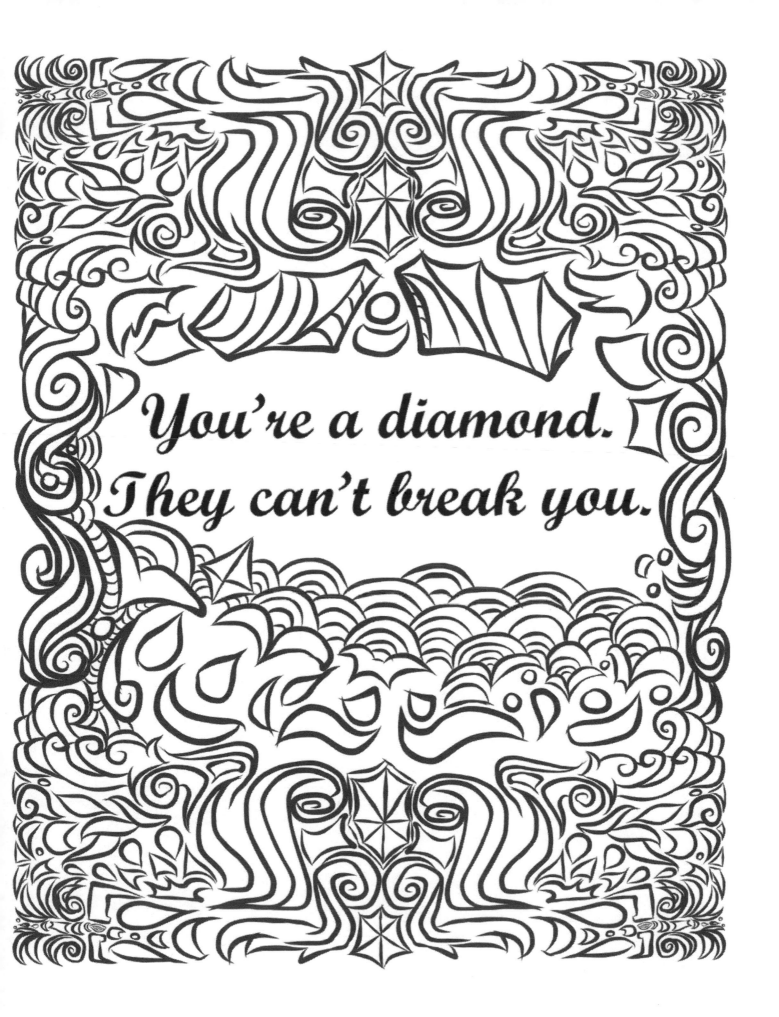

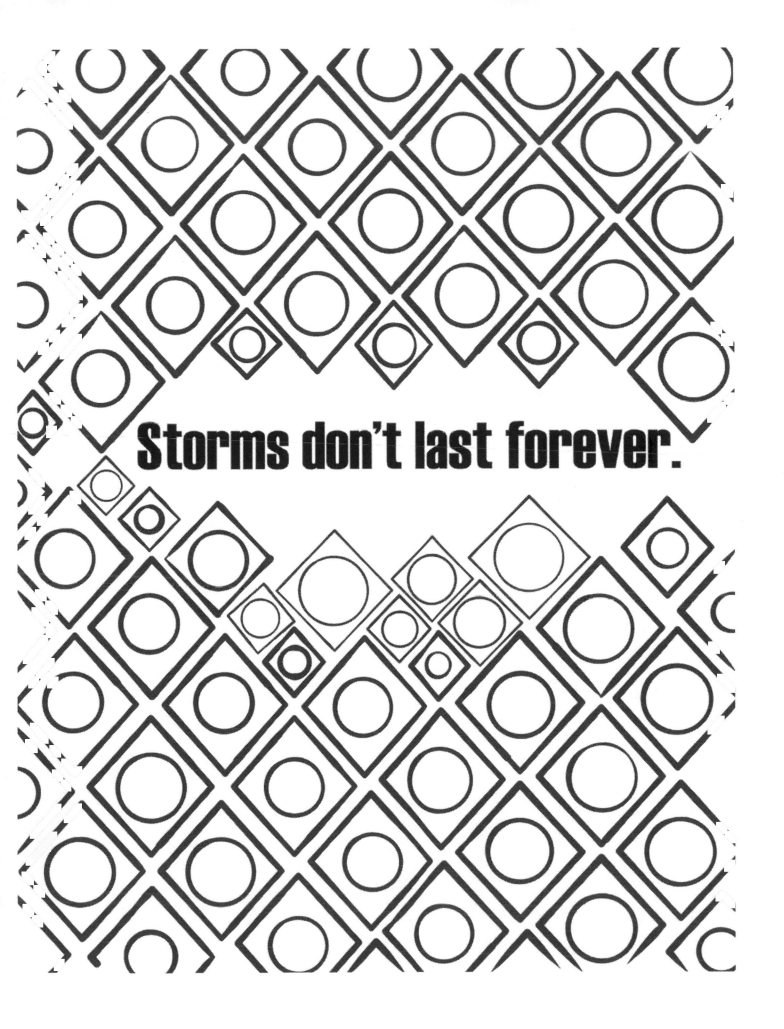

Storms don't last forever.

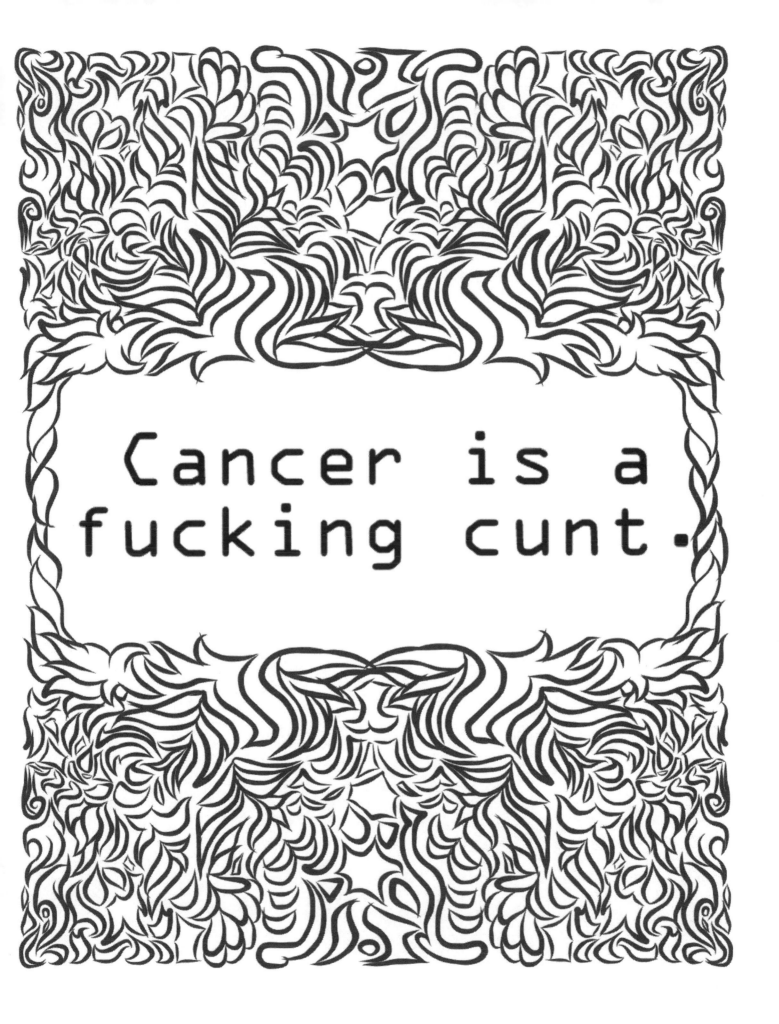

Cancer is a
fucking cunt.

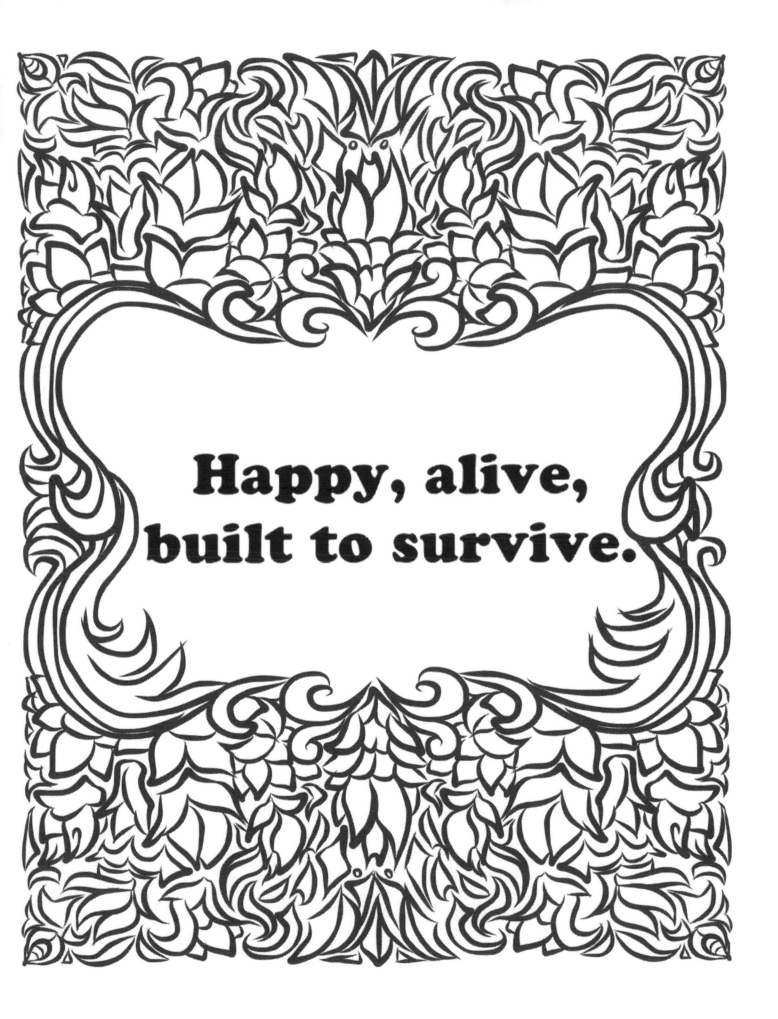

Happy, alive, built to survive.

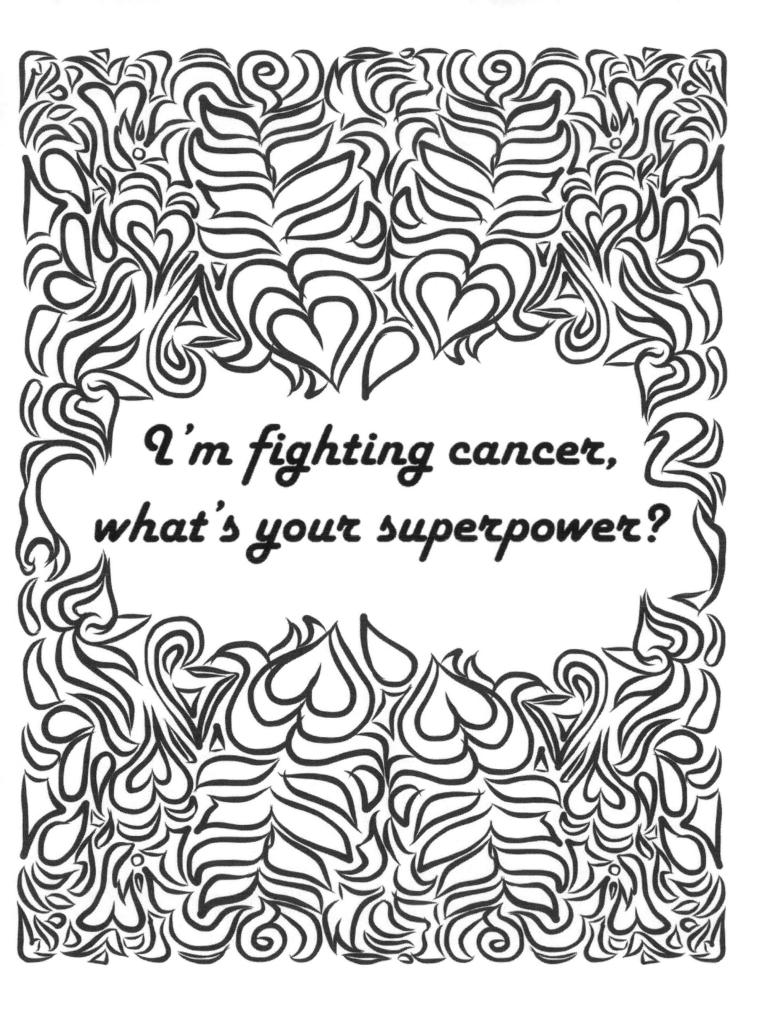

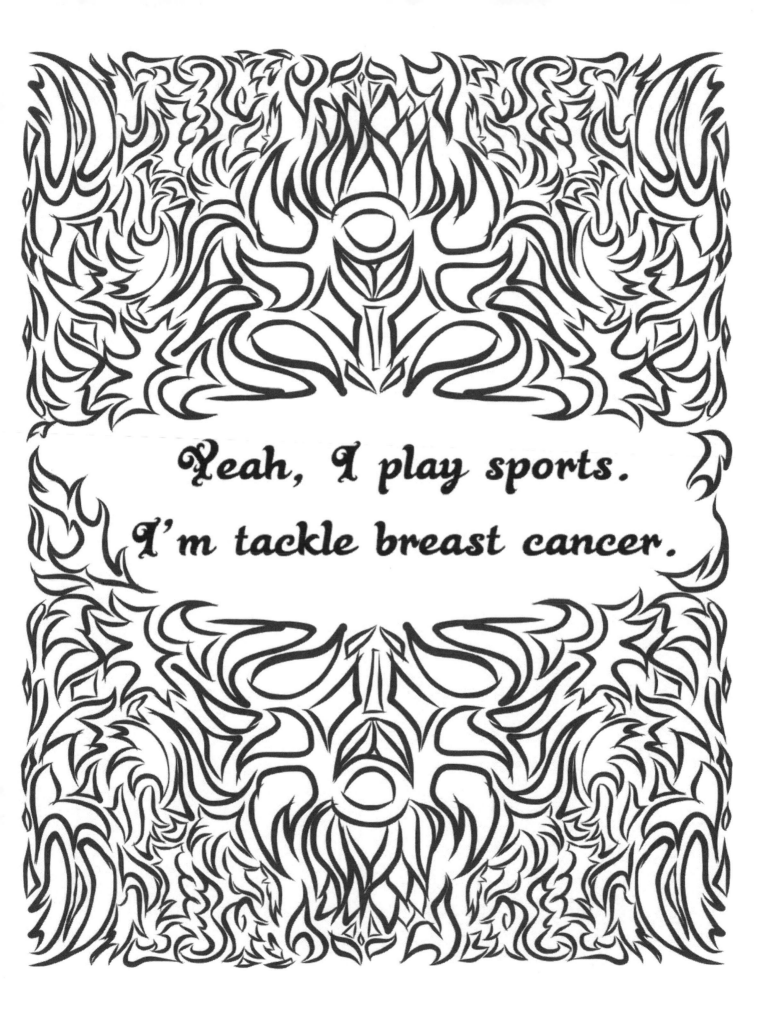

Yeah, I play sports.
I'm tackle breast cancer.

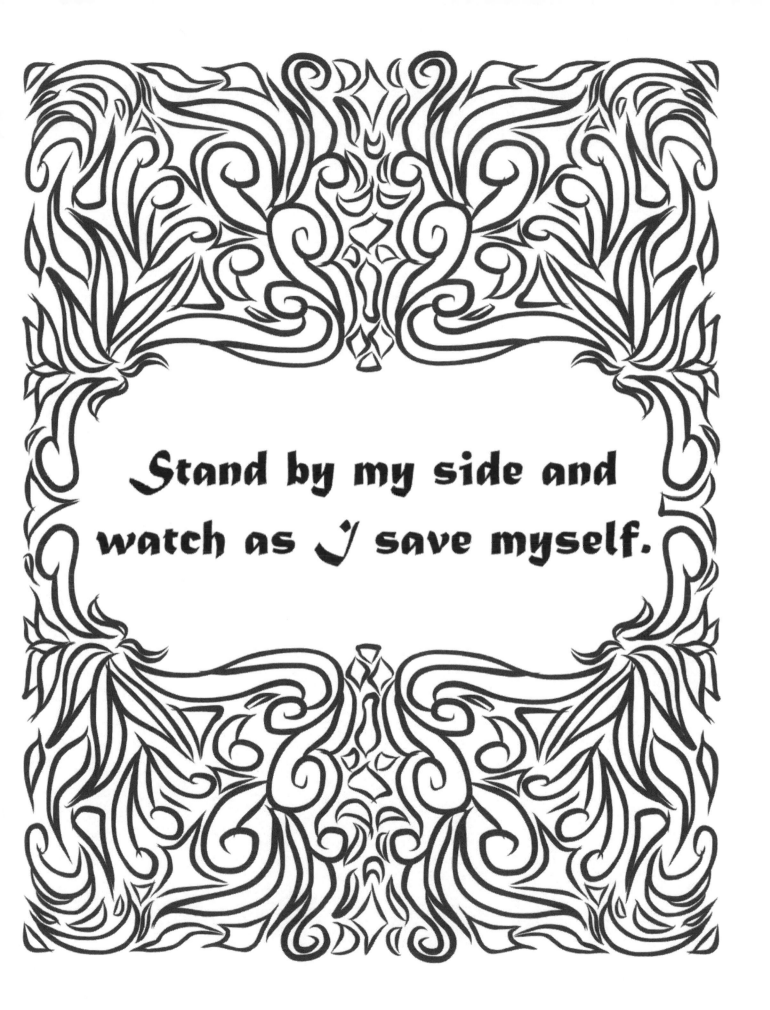

Stand by my side and watch as I save myself.

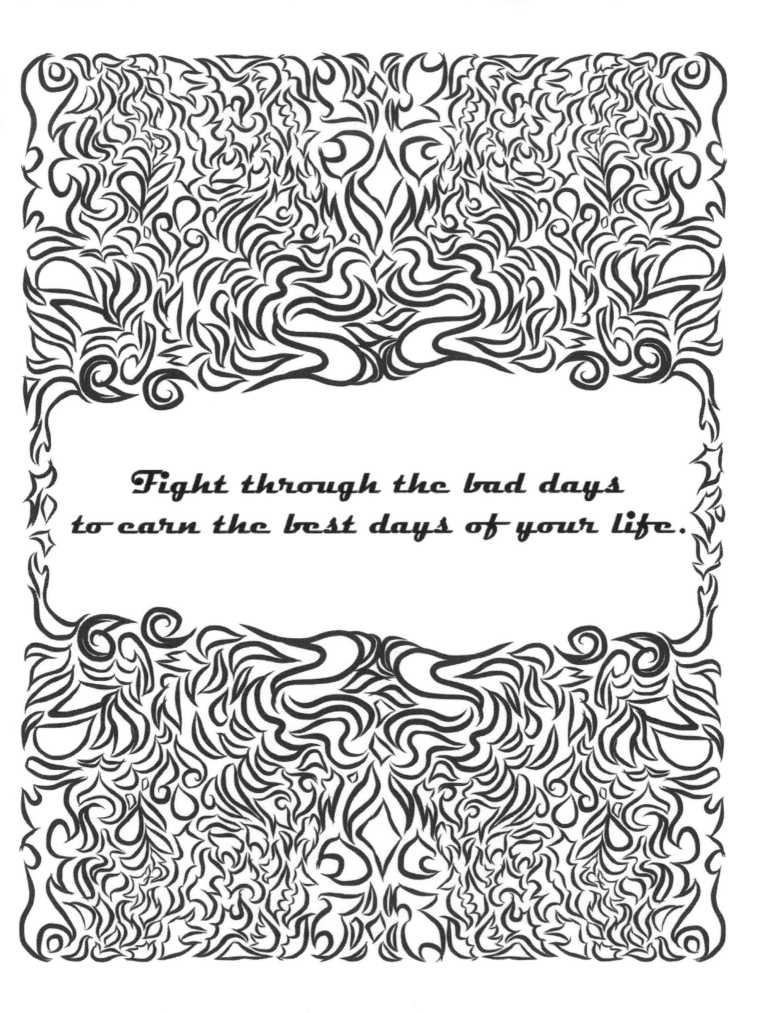

Fight through the bad days
to earn the best days of your life.

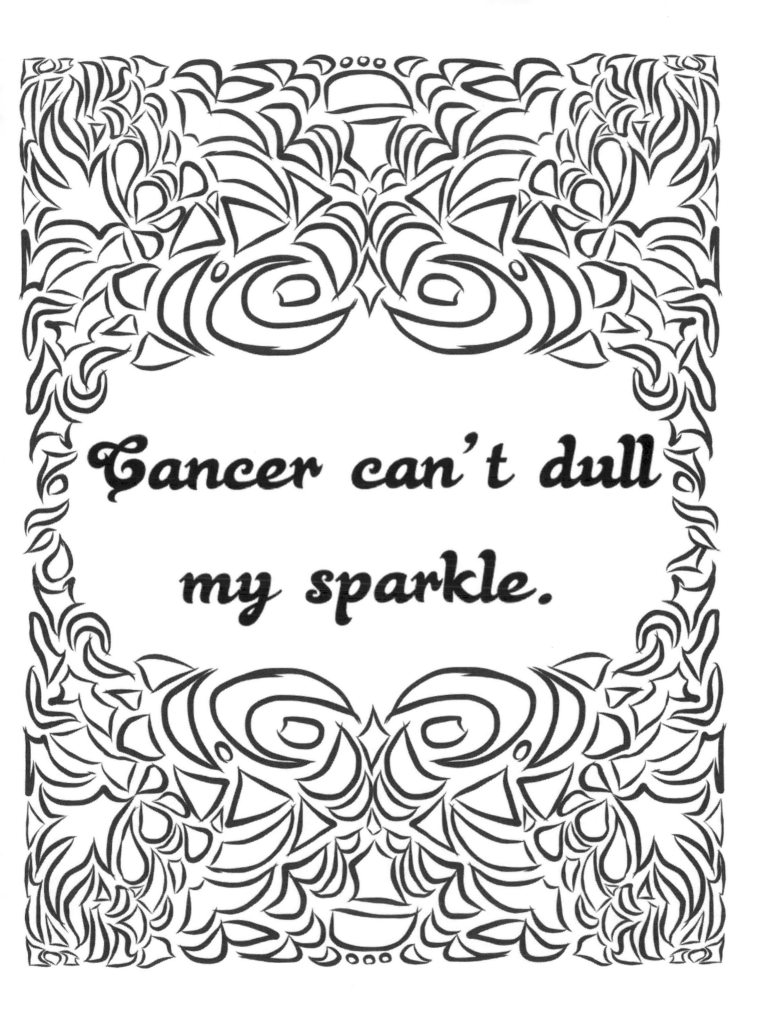

Cancer can't dull my sparkle.

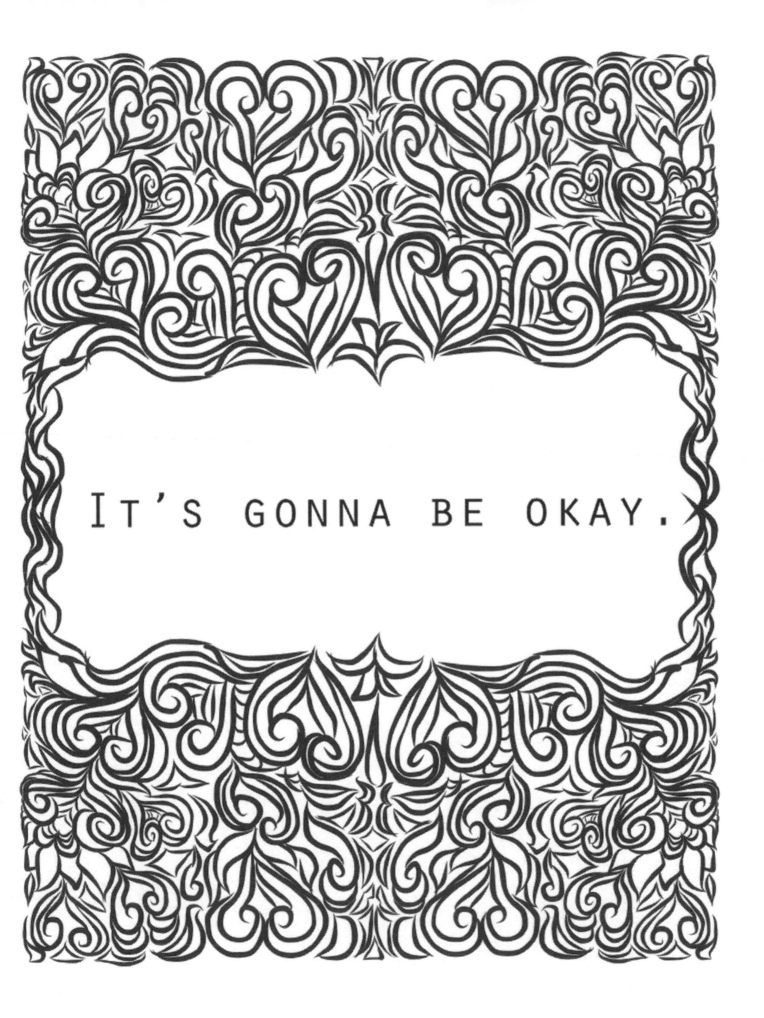

IT'S GONNA BE OKAY.

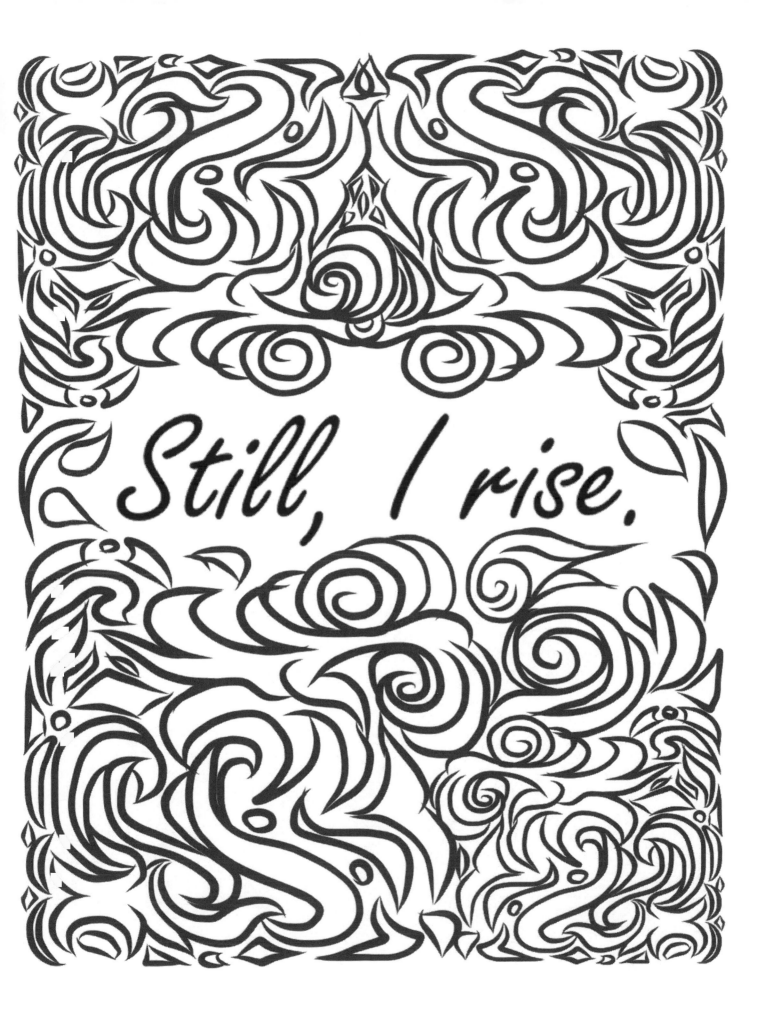

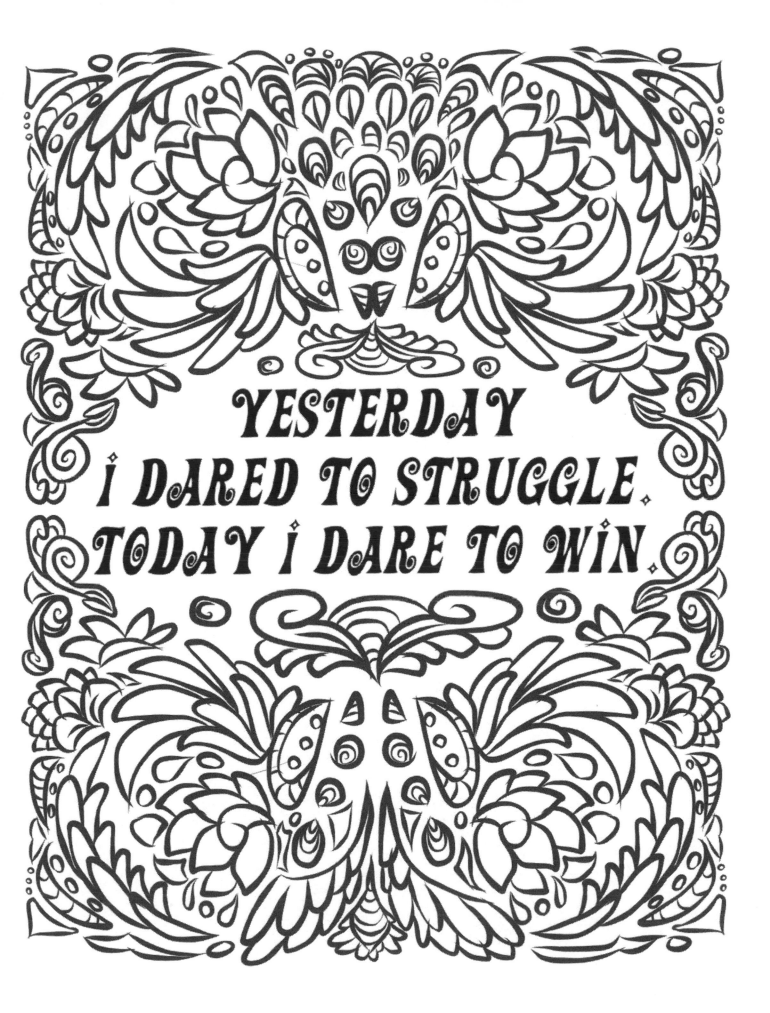

Thanks for purchasing and coloring this activity book!
If you enjoyed it, we'd love to hear what you loved most and what
you'd like to see in the future. Please consider taking a few minutes to
leave a review on Amazon. Being independent artists, it is only
with support from amazing people like yourself that
we are able to reach more people, share our work and build
an amazing community. Can't wait to create more amazing
work for you ☺

Thank you for your support,
Annie at Kingsley Publishing

WANT MORE GOODIES?

Join our email list here for **a free printable coloring book,** tons of freebies, giveaways, flash sale alerts and more fun!

http://bit.ly/GetFreeColoringBook

Want some printable fun? Visit us on Etsy:

Etsy.com/shop/KingsleyPublishing

Made in the USA
Monee, IL
10 September 2020